# Intermittent Fasting For Women Over 50

*A Complete Guide with All Secrets of Intermittent Fasting to Reduce Weight, Promote Longevity, and Better Heart Health, with Recipes for more than 365 Days and a 28-Day Meal Plan*

D1557165

**By**

**CAMILLE ROSE**

Respective authors own all copyrights not held by the publisher.

The information herein is offered for informational purposes solely and is universal as so. The presentation of the information is without a contract or any guarantee assurance. The trademarks that are used are without any consent, and the publication of the trademark is without permission or backing by the trademark owner. All trademarks and brands within this book are for clarifying purposes only and are owned by the owners themselves, not affiliated with this document.

# Table of Contents

# Introduction

Women over the age of 50 may encounter difficulties when attempting to lose weight. This can be due to a variety of factors. Often, the primary issue is a sluggish metabolism. Your metabolism will be faster if you have slimmer muscle. However, as we age, we lose lean muscle and frequently become less active than we were. As a result? Rigid body fat that simply would not go away.

Intermittent fasting has grown in popularity in recent years due to the variety of health benefits it provides and the fact that it does not restrict your dietary choices. Fasting has been shown to boost metabolism, psychological health and may even help avoid some malignancies. Additionally, it can help women over 50 avoid certain muscular, nerve, and joint issues.

Intermittent fasting has grown in popularity over the last few years.

Unlike most diets, which dictate what you should eat, intermittent fasting emphasizes when you should eat by including daily short-term fasts into your regimen.

This type of eating may assist you in consuming fewer calories, losing weight, and decreasing your chance of developing diabetes or heart disease.

Several studies, however, have indicated that intermittent fasting isn't quite as advantageous to women as it is to males. As a result, women may require a different approach.

This is a comprehensive guide to intermittent fasting for ladies over the age of 50.

# Chapter 1: Intermittent Fasting – The Basics and Types

## 1.1 What Is Intermittent Fasting?

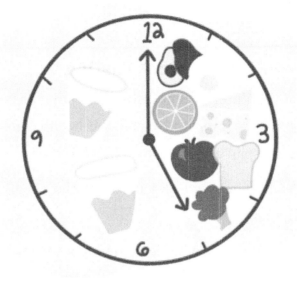

It is an eating plan that alternates between intervals of eating and fasting. IF is a type of intermittent fasting. However, it does not tell you what meals you should eat, but rather when.

In this regard, it's not a diet in the normal sense but rather an eating regimen. A common way of intermittent fasting is to go on a 16-hour fast once a day or a 24-hour fast twice weekly.

Humans have been practicing fasting since the beginning of time. There were no supermarkets, refrigerators, or year-round food supplies for ancient hunter-gatherers. They ran out of food on occasion.

Consequently, people have evolved to go without food for long periods without regaining consciousness. Rather than eating three or four times a day, it is more natural to fast from time to time. Fasting is a common practice in many religions, including Judaism, Christianity, Islam, and Buddhism, for spiritual or religious purposes.

## 1.2 Types Of Intermittent Fasting

It's no secret that intermittent fasting is a popular new health trend. Weight loss, improved metabolic health, and possibly an extended life span are all claimed by devotees.

Choosing the best method is a personal choice, and no two people are the same.

This eating pattern can be implemented in a variety of ways. It is important to consult a doctor before beginning an intermittent fast or determining how often to fast.

Six popular approaches to intermittent fasting are listed below.

### 1. The 5:2 diet

The 5:2 diet entails eating normally five days a week and lowering your calorie consumption to 500–600 calories on two days.

This diet is also known as the Fast Diet.

On fasting days, ladies should consume 500 calories, and males should consume 600.

For instance, you may normally eat on all days, excluding Mondays and Thursdays. You consume 2 minor meals of 250 calories each for ladies and 300 calories each for men during those two days.

This type of diet is beneficial for weight loss.

## 2. The 16/8 method

If you follow the 16/8 method, you'll fast for about 16 hours a day and only eat for about 8 hours each day. All meals can be consumed inside the dining window.

This method of fasting might be as simple as skipping breakfast and eating nothing after dinner. A 16-hour fast, for example, occurs when you quit eating at 8 pm and don't eat again until midday on the following day.

This method may take some time to adapt to people who are hungry in the morning and like breakfast. Although many people who skip breakfast do so regularly, this isn't always the case.

To reduce hunger pangs during fasting, you can consume water and coffee or other low-calorie beverages, such as herbal tea. Throughout your eating window, it is essential to eat healthily. If you eat a lot of processed food or calories, this technique won't work.

### 3. Eat Stop Eat

A 24-hour fast either once or twice a week is part of Eat Stop Eat. A 24-hour fast is achieved by fasting from supper one day to dinner the following day.

To put this in context, let's say you finish your meal at 7 pm Monday and don't eat again until 7 pm Tuesday, which is the end of your 24-hour fast. You can also fast from lunch to lunch, but the end outcome is the same.

During the fast, coffee, water, and other low-calorie liquids are tolerated, but solid food is not. To keep your weight in check, you must adhere to your normal diet while eating. You should consume the same quantity of the food as if you hadn't fasted at all.

A 24-hour fast may be a challenge for many people. Therefore this strategy may not be suitable for everyone. There is no need to jump in headfirst. A good starting point is between 14 and 16 hours.

### 4. The Warrior Diet

During the day, you eat small portions of raw vegetables and fruits, and at night, you consume a large dinner. Fasting all day and feasting at night inside a 4-hour window is basically how it works.

When the Warrior Diet originally came out, it was among the first popular diets incorporating intermittent fasting. Predominantly whole and unprocessed foods make up the bulk of this diet's dietary selections.

## 5. Alternate-Day Fasting

Fasting every other day is called alternate-day fasting. There are a variety of ways to implement this strategy. During the days of fasting, some of them enable roughly 500 calories to be consumed by the body.

Small studies show that alternate-day fasting is no more effective than a regular calorie-restrictive diet for weight loss and maintenance. If you're new to fasting, a full fast every day is not recommended.

Using this strategy, you may find yourself going to bed several hungry nights a week, which is not pleasant and is probably not sustainable in the long term.

## 6. Spontaneous Meal Skipping

To get some of the benefits of intermittent fasting, you don't need to adhere to a predetermined regimen. You can skip meals if you don't feel like eating or are too occupied with cooking and eating.

On the other hand, some people frequently eat to avoid going into starvation mode or losing muscle. Other people's bodies are well-equipped to tolerate prolonged famine and can go a few days without food without harming their health. You're the only one who knows you.

So, if you don't feel like eating breakfast on a given day, you may simply eat a nutritious lunch and dinner instead. Some people choose to go on a fast when they are on the road because they can't find food they like while they are there. When you skip a meal or two whenever you feel like it, you're simply engaging in an intermittent fast.

During the non-fasting periods, make sure to consume nutritious, balanced meals.

## 1.3 Health Benefits Of Intermittent Fasting

Having a better understanding of the health benefits of intermittent fasting can help you get motivated to give it a try. To be truly powerful, one must have access to as much information as possible. However, fat loss isn't the sole advantage of fasting.

### 1. Your day is made easier by intermittent fasting.

Behavior modification, simplification, and stress reduction are all important to me. For me, the additional simplicity that intermittent fasting brings to my life is a huge plus. I don't think about breakfast when I wake up. To begin my day, I simply pour myself a drink of water and go about my business.

Having 3 meals a day was never a chore for me because I enjoy it, and I don't mind cooking. Fasting on an intermittent basis, on the other hand, has allowed me to cut down on the number of meals I have to prepare and arrange each day. It makes life a little easier for me, which is a positive thing.

## 2. If you want to live a longer life, try intermittent fasting.

Scientists have known for a long time that cutting back on calories can help you live longer. This makes sense from a logical standpoint. Our bodies have a way of extending our lives when we're hungry.

Only one issue stands in the way: Who would willingly starve oneself to live longer?

You may not share my desire for long life, but I do. It doesn't sound all that appealing to go on a hunger strike.

The great news is that fasting stimulates most of the same processes as calorie restriction to lengthen lifespan. As a result, you reap the benefits of a long life span without having to worry about starving yourself to death in the process.

In 1945, intermittent fasting was discovered to extend the lives of mice. Intermittent fasting on alternate days may lengthen one's life span, according to a recent study.

### 3. Cancer risk may be reduced by intermittent fasting.

There hasn't been a lot of research into the connection between cancer and fasting, so this one is up for debate. However, early indications are encouraging.

According to a study of ten cancer patients, fasting before chemotherapy may lessen the negative effects. Fasting before chemotherapy improved cure rates and decreased mortality, according to a separate trial that included cancer patients on alternate-day fasting.

A recent review of numerous studies on intermittent fasting and sickness has found that it may help prevent cancer and heart disease.

### 4. When it comes to dieting, intermittent fasting is a lot easier.

Most diets fail because people don't stick with them long enough, not because they employ the wrong foods. No, the issue isn't one of nourishment; rather, it is one of behavioral change.

As soon as you get over the assumption that you have to constantly consume food, intermittent fasting becomes a viable option. "Subjects quickly adapt" to a pattern of intermittent fasting, according to a study that found it to be a successful technique for losing weight in obese individuals.

The idea of going on a diet has crossed our minds many times. When we find a diet that we enjoy, sticking to it becomes second nature. However, when we get down to the nitty-gritty, it gets difficult.

There is no doubt that intermittent fasting is difficult to contemplate. When I described what I was doing, folks were bewildered and said, "You mean you don't eat?" "I'd never be able to accomplish that," I said. However, once you get going, it's a cinch. For one or two of the 3 meals a day, there are no concerns about what to eat or where to dine. It's a wonderful feeling of freedom to be able to do this. Expenditures on food fall precipitously. And you don't appear to be in the mood to eat. ... Although it's difficult to get over the concept of going without eating, nothing could be simpler once you start the regimen."

Other benefits include:

- Diabetes Control: There is evidence that fasting helps lower one's diabetes risk. As a result of the lower insulin levels, the body does not have to work as hard to keep glucose levels stable while fasting.

- Low blood pressure and lower LDL cholesterol are linked to improved cardiovascular health.

- When insulin levels are reduced, stored fat can be utilized as energy, leading to weight loss.

- Reduced Inflammation: Eating does not lessen inflammation in the body. The kidneys can better remove extra salt and water from the body when there is less insulin in the blood. This reduces inflammation.

- Growth Hormone levels rise, resulting in increased muscle mass. Your lean muscle mass increases while you fast and work out at the same time. A greater number of calories are burned when you have a greater number of muscles.

- Reduced Blood Pressure: When excess water and salt are flushed from the kidneys, blood pressure levels are lower.

- An increase in metabolism is a natural side effect of elevated levels of adrenalin.

- Fasting has been shown to increase one's psychological well-being, including a better perception of one's own body and less despair.

- You can naturally minimize your calorie intake by not eating outside of the fasting window when you're fasting.

- Improved Cognitive Function: When you embark on a fasting regimen, your mental acuity and clarity improve.

- Cell regeneration and improved function are two benefits of fasting that can help you live a longer, healthier life.

## 1.4 A Highly Effective Weight-Reduction Tool

Intermittent fasting is most commonly used to lose weight. Intermittent fasting might reduce your calorie consumption by having you eat fewer meals. Intermittent fasting also alters hormone levels, which aids in weight loss, as well. While insulin and growth hormone are reduced, the fat-burning hormone norepinephrine is increased (noradrenaline).

Short-term fasting may raise your metabolic rate by 3.6–14% because of these hormonal changes. Intermittent fasting affects weight reduction by altering both parts of the calorie equation: eating less and exercising more. Intermittent fasting is a powerful weight loss strategy. Relative to most weight-reduction research, a 2014 analysis indicated that this way of eating could result in 3–8 percent weight loss over 3–24 weeks.

In the same study, people also dropped between 4–7 percent of their waist circumference, which indicates a considerable reduction in the dangerous belly fat that accumulates surrounding your organs and causes sickness.

In another study, it was found that intermittent fasting results in less muscle loss than calorie-restricted diets.

It's important to bear in mind, though, that the fundamental reason for its popularity is that intermittent fasting makes you consume fewer overall calories. You may not lose any weight if you eat a lot throughout your eating times and binge on junk food.

## 1.5 Maintaining a Healthy Lifestyle Is Now Easier

While eating healthy is straightforward, it can be exceedingly difficult to maintain. One of the primary impediments is the amount of work needed to plan and prepare healthy meals. Intermittent fasting can simplify things, as it eliminates the need to plan, cook, and tidy up after as numerous meals as previously required.

As a result, intermittent fasting is quite popular within the life-hacking community, as it enhances your health while also simplifying your life.

## 1.6 Foods That Are Allowed During Intermittent Fasting

Before making any big changes to your diet, consider a health professional to ensure the change is right for you.

There are no requirements or restrictions on the type or quantity of food consumed during intermittent fasting.

You may drink water or zero-calorie liquids such as black tea or coffee when you are not eating.

And "eating normally" during your eating intervals does not entail going insane. If you stuff your mealtimes with greater calorie junk food, fried foods, and snacks, you're unlikely to lose weight or improve your health.

Consume a variety of the following foods to avoid developing hangry anger when fasting.

## 1. Avacado

Consuming the greatest fruit while attempting to reduce weight may seem paradoxical. Avocados, on the other hand, owing to their high unsaturated fat content, will keep you satisfied during even the most stringent fasting periods.

Unsaturated fats, according to research, keep the body content even when you don't feel full. Your body communicates that it has sufficient nourishment and is not about to enter emergency famine mode. Unsaturated fats prolong these indications, even if you feel a little hungry during a fasting period.

Another study discovered that including half an avocado in your lunch may help you feel fuller for hours extra than if you skip the green, mushy treasure.

## 2. Drinking Water

While this is not exactly food, it is critical for surviving IF. Water plays a critical role in the health of virtually every major organ in your body. You would be unwise to exclude this from your fast. Your organs are critical for, well, being alive.

The amount of water that each individual should drink varies according to their gender, height, weight, degree of exercise, and climate. However, the color of your urine is a good indicator. At all times, you would like it to be pale yellow.

Dark yellow urine indicates dehydration, which can manifest itself in the form of headaches, weariness, and lightheadedness. Combine this with a scarcity of food, and you have a dangerous mix — or, at the very worst, extremely dark pee.

If plain water does not appeal to you, try adding a few fresh mints, a squeeze of lemon, or some cucumber slices to it.

### 3. Seafood And Fish

There is a reason why the American Dietary Guidelines recommend 2 to 3 four-ounce portions of fish per week. Along with being rich in healthy fats and protein, it is a good source of vitamin D.

And if eating at restricted times is your thing, don't you want to get the most nutritional value for your money when you eat?

There are so many different methods to prepare fish that you will never get out of inspiration.

## 4. Potatoes

In the 1990s, the researchers discovered that potatoes were among the most satiating foods. Additionally, a 2012 study discovered that including potatoes in a balanced diet may aid in

weight loss. Regrettably, potato chips and french fries do not qualify.

## 5. Cruciferous Plants And Vegetables

Fiber-rich foods include brussels sprouts, broccoli, and cauliflower. When eating at regular intervals, it is critical to consume fiber-rich meals to keep you regular and your poop factory running efficiently.

Additionally, fiber might help you feel full, which may be beneficial if you cannot eat for 16 hours. Cruciferous vegetables may also help lessen your risk of cancer.

## 6. Legumes And Beans

Food, specifically carbohydrate-containing foods, provides energy for action. We're not advocating carbohydrate overload, but it certainly wouldn't harm to incorporate some low-calorie carbs like legumes and beans into your diet. This can help you maintain a positive attitude throughout your fasting hours.

Additionally, foods such as chickpeas, peas, black beans, and lentils have been demonstrated to help people lose weight even when they are not on a calorie-restricted diet.

## 7. Berries

These smoothie essentials are nutrient-dense. And it isn't even the most amazing part.

According to a 2016 study, persons who ingested a large number of flavonoids, such as those present in strawberries and blueberries, had lower BMI rises over 14 years than those who did not consume berries.

## 8. Probiotics

What do the small organisms in your gut prefer? Consistency and variation. That is, they are not content when they are hungry. Additionally, if your gut is unhappy, you may encounter unpleasant side effects, such as constipation.

To combat this discomfort, incorporate probiotic-rich foods into your diet, including kefir, kombucha, and sauerkraut.

## 9. Eggs

One big egg has 6.24 grams of protein and takes only minutes to cook. And consuming as much protein as necessary is critical for maintaining a healthy weight and muscle growth, even more so when eating less.

According to a 2010 study, males who ate an egg breakfast rather than a bagel have been less hungry and consumed less food throughout the day.

In other words, if you're bored during your period of fasting, why not hard-boil some eggs? Then, when the moment is appropriate, you can eat them.

## 10. Whole Grains

Consuming carbs while on a diet appears to fall into two distinct categories. You will be ecstatic to learn that this is not always the case. Whole grains are high in fiber and protein, so a small amount will keep you satisfied.

Therefore, push yourself out of your comfort bubble and into a whole-grain utopia composed of bulgur, farro, spelled, sorghum, amaranth, Kamut, millet, or freekeh.

## 11. Nuts

While nuts include more calories than other snacks, they provide something that other snack items do not: healthy fats.

Additionally, if you're concerned about calories, have no fear! According to a 2012 study, a 1-ounce portion of almonds (approximately 23 nuts) contains 20% fewer calories than the label indicates. According to a study, gnawing does not entirely dissolve the cell walls of almonds. This preserves a part of the nut and prevents it from being absorbed by the body during digestion. As a result, if you consume almonds, they may not make as much of a hole in your everyday calorie intake as you believed.

## 12. Hummus

Hummus, one of the creamiest and most delectable dips known to humanity, is another wonderful source of plant-based protein and an ideal method to enhance the nutrient quality of

staples like sandwiches—simply substitute it for mayonnaise. If you're confident enough to prepare your hummus, keep in mind that the optimal recipe requires garlic and tahini.

## 13. Seitan

One significant investigation established a direct correlation between red meat consumption and higher mortality. Utilize your anti-aging fast to its full potential by consuming life-extending plant-based protein alternatives such as seitan. This delicacy, often known as "wheat meat," can be baked, battered, or dipped in your favorite sauces.

## 14. Multivitamin Supplements

One potential theory for IF results in weight loss are that the individual has so little time to eat and hence consumes less food. While the notion of energy in versus energy out is accurate, what is sometimes overlooked is the risk of vitamin shortages while on a caloric deficit. While a multivitamin is not required if you eat a balanced diet rich in vegetables and fruits, life may get hectic, and a supplement can assist fill in the gaps.

## 15. Vitamin D Fortified Milk

The recommended daily calcium intake for an adult is 1,000 milligrams or roughly three glasses of milk. With a smaller eating window, chances to drink this amount may be limited, which is why it is critical to emphasize calcium-rich foods. Vitamin D enriched milk improves the body's calcium

absorption and helps maintain strong bones. You can add milk to cereals or smoothies or drink it with meals to increase your calcium consumption daily. If you're not a lover of the beverage, other calcium-rich non-dairy options include soy products and tofu, as well as leafy green vegetables like kale.

## 16. Papaya

During the last hours of your fast, you're likely to experience hunger symptoms, especially if you're new to intermittent fasting. This "hanger" may then lead to binge eating, leaving you bloated and tired minutes later. Papaya has a unique enzyme called papain, which degrades proteins. By using slices of this tropical fruit in a protein-rich meal, you can aid digestion and manage any bloat.

## 17. Salad Dressing Made at Home

Just as your grandma kept her cuisine basic and wholesome, you should keep salad sauces and dressings simple and wholesome as well. When we prepare our basic dressings, we avoid unnecessary additives and added sugar.

## 1.7 Is Intermittent Fasting Safe?

Irritable bowel syndrome (IBS), high cholesterol (LDL), and arthritis are chronic illnesses that can benefit from intermittent fasting. It's not for everyone, however.

It's best to consult with your primary care physician before starting any diet, including intermittent fasting. Intermittent fasting may not be right for everyone:

- Minors and young adults under the age of 18

- Breastfeeding or expecting mothers.

- People with diabetes and those with blood sugar issues.

- As well as those who have previously suffered from an eating issue.

In the absence of these conditions, those who can safely adhere to intermittent fasting can do so for as long as they like. As she puts it, "It may be a lifestyle shift, and one that has advantages."

The consequences of intermittent fasting can vary from person to person. If you begin to experience unusual anxiety, nausea, headaches, or other symptoms after an intermittent fasting regimen, you should consult your physician.

## 1.8 How Does Intermittent Fasting Work?

Intermittent fasting can be done in various methods, but they all revolve around establishing a regular eating and fasting schedule. You could, for example, eat only for eight hours of the day and fast for the rest of the time. If you choose, you can have only 1 meal a day for 2 days a week. Intermittent fasting has a variety of schedules.

Intermittent fasting is a radical departure from the typical American eating pattern, in which most people eat throughout the day. They are running on calories and not utilizing their fat stores every time they consume three or more meals a day, and not exercising. Your body burns through the calories you ate after your last meal and starts burning fat when you go on an intermittent fast.

## 1.9 What Happens To Women Body Over 50

New, stronger bone cells are replaced with older ones as you get older. Over time, the number of broken-down bone cells in your body exceeds the number of new bone cells that can be created. Bones naturally weaken over time.

## 1.10 Tips And Common Mistakes To Avoid When Intermittent Fasting For Women

Fasting is easier if you keep these things in mind to help ease the transition.

- Shorten your workouts if you start to feel dizzy or dizzy when you're fasting, or take a break and come back to it the next day if you've had an off day.

- At all times, keep your body hydrated.

- Eat a balanced diet that includes plenty of protein, healthy fats, fiber, and complex carbs.

- To ensure that your meals don't just include empty calories, stay away from processed foods.

- When fasting, use a baking soda solution instead of toothpaste, and avoid drugs like Advil with a sugar coating.

# Chapter 2: Getting Started on IF

## 2.1 How To Start Intermittent Fasting For Women?

Nice to hear. Intermittent Fasting is simple to get started with, and there are only two rules to remember.

Make sure to drink enough water before beginning a fast to avoid migraines and hunger as you get used to lasting long periods without food. Add 1 to 2 tsp of apple cider vinegar to your water if you are experiencing hunger pangs. In addition to reducing appetite, it has been shown to aid in weight loss. In addition, if you're fasting, don't eat. That's the second simple guideline to remember.

Try to keep things as simple as possible. To begin, try going without eating for several hours to observe how you feel. Skip one meal and gradually increase to two. Make it a point to eat healthfully whenever possible so that you can enjoy your life to the fullest.

Before embarking on an IF regimen, consult your doctor. When making major lifestyle changes, such as changing your diet or exercising, acquire a medical clearance first.

## 2.2 Why Start Intermittent Fasting Over 50?

For women over 50, intermittent fasting may lead to weight loss and reduce the risk of acquiring age-related diseases. According to a new study of Medicine, intermittent fasting can decrease blood pressure. According to the study, fasting reduces blood pressure by altering the bacteria in one's gut.

In addition to their desire to better their health, many women over 50 are concerned about losing weight. As we get older, our metabolism slows, our joints ache, our muscle mass decreases, and our ability to get a good night's sleep diminishes. However, shedding pounds, particularly harmful abdominal fat, can significantly lower your chance of developing diabetes, heart disease, and cancer.

Many diseases are more likely to occur as you get older. Some women over the age of 50 may benefit from intermittent fasting in weight loss and reducing their risk of acquiring age-related disorders.

Nutritionists are divided on whether or not intermittent fasting (IF) is effective since it encourages people to eat fewer calories than they would otherwise consume. With the same caloric intake and other nutrients, they consider that intermittent fasting effects are superior. Many studies have shown that refraining from food for a few hours per day does more than merely reduce the number of calories you eat each day.

IF has several metabolic alterations that may explain synergistic effects:

- Lower levels of insulin during the period of fasting aid fat loss.

- HGH: As insulin levels decrease, HGH levels increase, promoting fat loss and muscle building.

- Noradrenaline: The nervous system sends this chemical to cells to inform them that they must release fat for fuel in response to an empty stomach.

## 2.3 Step-By-Step Starting Approach

### Step 1: Remove Breakfast off the Plate

Cutting off breakfast is the simplest and most effective approach to begin intermittent fasting. In the morning, your body does its own thing. Food is merely a stumbling block. The adrenals and cortisol chemicals increase in the morning to help you awaken, become awake, and generate energy.

Fasting is a great way to take advantage of your body's natural circadian rhythms.

### Step 2: Determine the Best Time of Day to Exercise

Many individuals mistakenly believe that they cannot exercise during fasting, but this is not the case. Exercise in the morning is the most efficient time of day! You've just woken up, and your hormones have been optimized.

Evening and afternoon workouts aren't usually the most successful because you're exhausted from the day, distracted by whatever new pressures fell in your lap at the office, and unable to resist the impulse to slip off your boots and decompress.

I stuck with my afternoon training regimen for more than a decade, but shifting to a morning hours' gym plan has been a game-changer. If I don't work out first thing in the morning, I can almost see the sliding scale as I miss out on opportunities for a quality workout during the day. As life grows hectic, so does one's energy level!

**Step 3: Calm down. Unsweetened coffee can still be enjoyed!**

Your voice is trembling with nervousness as you inquire, "Can I drink coffee while I'm fasting?"

Yes! Fortunately for coffee consumers everywhere, our beloved morning habit does not raise blood sugar levels or disturb your fast.

If you don't like the taste of black coffee, you can always add a little creamer to it. Just a little bit, please! Remember that before your body can resume burning your stored fat, it must first burn thru the fat in the creamer.

For those who prefer their coffee sweetened, what about those who prefer it without? All-natural sweeteners, such as honey, cane sugar, and agave nectar should be avoided. They may be "natural," but the spike in insulin and blood sugar they cause is anything but. As a result, your body is no longer in a fasting state.

Use only a small amount of Stevia in your coffee if you want it to be a little sweeter. Artificial sugars are harmful because they trigger cravings and deceive your digestive system into thinking it's about to receive sugar. Fasting's intended fat-burning effect is seriously jeopardized if this happens.

It all comes down to what you want to accomplish. Using a cream to your morning coffee may hinder your weight loss efforts if you're trying to shed 50 pounds. However, a piece of cheesecake is no match for a cup of sweet coffee! It's all about finding a middle ground.

## Step 4: This Is For Diabetics, Too!

Intermittent fasting is an effective strategy to lower and regulate blood sugar levels in people with type 2 diabetes, a disease characterized by increased amounts of blood sugar.

Fasting is one of the most effective strategies I recommend to my patients to help them achieve better glycemic control. It's possible that people with diabetes can use fasting to reduce their reliance on medicine and lessen the consequences of their condition by following a well-planned strategy under the guidance of their doctor.

## Step 5: Plan Your Meals Based On The Fasting Cycles

Now that you've heard it all, you're ready to jump into the lovely world of intermittent fasting. Congratulations. So, when exactly are you allowed to consume food?

It's easiest to forgo breakfast in favor of a cup of coffee or tea. Eat a low-carb dinner and lunch if you want to lose weight.

As soon as your fasting window closes, you'll have six to eight hours to consume all you want to eat for the day.

That's a matter of opinion. Make it fit into your daily routine... Great if it's six hours. Don't feel bad if you have to work into the wee hours of the morning.

There is no right or wrong when it comes to intermittent fasting. It's a technique to enhance your health in a way that works with your daily schedule.

## Step 6: Join The Dinnertime Crowd

Breakfast is the most important meal of the day, and most people skip it. Our dinners provide a chance for us to get to know one other better. It's been like this from the beginning of time! At dinner, we utilize it as a time to unwind after a long day and reunite with our loved ones. The richness of the experience doesn't have to be denied to you.

Instead, make use of the chance to cultivate a state of attentive eating. You'll savor every mouthful of your dinner more than if you'd been munching all day long. Dinner is the most important meal of the day when it comes to fasting.

## Step 7: Consume Food That Is Suitable For Your Purpose

During intermittent fasting, we've figured out when to open our mouths. However, what exactly should you eat when you open your mouth? If you're looking to achieve a certain goal, there is no one-size-fits-all option.

### To lose weight, you should:

You can lose weight while fasting by decreasing the number of carbohydrates and sugars you consume. Breaking your fast should be as simple as possible, so schedule your meals ahead of time. Preparing a nutritious, low-carb lunch will help you avoid impulsive decisions. Don't break your fast if Burger King is the only option around.

For dinner, it's best to have lean protein and vegetables with a healthy carbohydrate or fat. In other words, eat things that nourish and fulfill you as a treat, not as punishment!

### If Weight Loss Isn't Your Biggest Priority!

Eating actual foods while fasting for health and longevity is the best strategy. Everything we eat today wasn't food a century ago. So, if you want to avoid the hidden sugar trap, stay away from processed, packaged goods and read labels carefully.

Proteins, good fats, and vegetables are the key to a nutritious diet. When you eat these genuine foods, you'll be able to limit your carbohydrate consumption without even realizing it.

The eighth step is to experiment with 24-hour fasting one day every week for one week.

Don't worry too much about the 24-hour fasting period. Is 24-hour fasting one day a week a major leap from intermittent fasting? Probably not.

After dinner, it is most convenient to begin a 24-hour fasting period. Instead of eating lunch at 1:00 in the afternoon, wait until night to break your fast.

If you've ever fasted for 24 hours, you'll know how gratifying it is to have your first meal after that. It's like nothing else. Additionally, giving your body a 24-hour recharge will help you burn fat and improve your biochemistry.

## Step 9: Avoiding Intermittent Fasting Cheat Days

Although binge days are similar in many respects to "cheat" days, they don't go away in a day or two for most people. After a cheat day, you may need 3 or 4 days to get back on track, rein in your desires, and regain your focus and energy.

What good is it to eat an entire pizza or a stack of pancakes if you're trying to lose weight? Having a cheat day where you eat 1,500 calories of junk food will have the opposite effect on your weight loss goals.

An indulgence, on the other hand, is a different matter. You can soothe an itch with a slice of pie or a few cookies now and again to prevent it from becoming a full-blown rash.

## 2.4 Intermittent Fasting And Sleep

Intermittent fasting may enhance your sleep quality by boosting your circadian cycles, according to research. Biological activities such as appetite, metabolism, and sleep-wake cycles are all controlled by your circadian rhythms. Sunlight is the primary circadian zeitgeber, or "time cue," for these processes, but the food is an important secondary zeitgeber. Fasting can help you maintain your natural circadian rhythms by following a strict food schedule.

Human growth hormone levels are higher in those who fast intermittently. This hormone, released during sleep, helps the body burn fat, build muscle, and repair itself at the cellular level. Consequently, fasting may result in a more rejuvenated and rejuvenated person when they wake up.

Intermittent fasting participants may also feel an increase in energy and attention. Orexin-A, a neurotransmitter linked to alertness, is increased during fasting. Fasters, in particular, have lower nighttime orexin-A levels and greater daytime orexin-A levels, allowing them to be more awake during the day and sleep better at night.

Intermittent fasting can have a positive impact on sleep in as little as a week. Intermittent fasting for a week improves sleep quality in healthy adults, according to a recent study. A more restful night's sleep was achieved because they were less prone to awaken in the night and slept more soundly. They also spent longer in rapid eye movement (REM) sleep, which is the stage of processing emotions and thoughts. They felt happier and more alert during the day due to the treatment, which improved their sleep, mood, and ability to concentrate.

## Hunger Can Affect Sleep

While we sleep, our bodies can control our hunger levels to some extent. As we sleep, leptin, the hormone that makes people feel full, rises in our bodies. Since leptin levels increase during intermittent fasting, you may not feel hungry for as long as you normally would.

Even if you eat dinner or a snack right before you go to bed, since sleep slows the appetite, you're in a similar situation when it comes to sleeping.

There are very few studies on fasting and the duration or quality of sleep in people. Therefore this is an area that needs more research. And there is no conclusive proof that fasting affects sleep or the other way around.

According to a new study, alternate-day fasting and time-restricted eating (when eating is limited to a specific period of time each day) do not have a significant impact on sleep.

Intermittent fasting does not appear to adversely affect sleep quality in the scientific literature.

**Insomnia Associated with Intermittent Fasting**

Even though intermittent fasting seems to increase sleep quality, the scheduling of your meals could lead to sleep problems. When people eat at odd hours, their sleep can be disrupted. This is particularly true if they dine late at night, which can boost the body's temperature, the exact reverse of what happens during a normal night's rest. The quality of your sleep and how rested you feel in the morning can both be harmed by eating large meals close to bedtime.

For example, fasting during Ramadan, in which you abstain from food during daylight hours and eat at night, interferes with your body's normal circadian cycles. A lack of melatonin is a sleep hormone, and less time in REM sleep may result from this conflict.

**While Fasting, These Tips Can Help You Get A Good Night's Sleep**

Maintaining a regular eating pattern may help you get a better night's sleep. A few good sleep habits will help you get a better night's rest while you're fasting.

**Do Not Go To Sleep Hungry**

A growling stomach can make it tough to drift off to sleep. Cortisol, a stress hormone, is released when you're hungry, which might affect your sleep quality.

Your last meal should be at least 3 hours away from bedtime. The digestion won't be disturbed while you sleep, but you won't go to bed hungry, either. This is an excellent compromise.

**Stay Hydrated**

Dehydration before going to sleep can lead to a less restful night's sleep. In addition to reducing your hunger pangs, drinking extra water during the day can help you sleep better at night.

Make sure you're not overdosing on caffeine and alcohol as well. Caffeine might help you lose weight, but it can also keep you up at night. In addition to affecting your metabolism and producing nutritional insufficiency, alcohol also interrupts sleep.

**Foods That Are Good for You**

Avoid foods high in glucose and empty calories, such as fast food and other processed foods. Keeping to a diet rich in nutrients will make it easier to stick to your intermittent fasting plan. Get your protein and lipids from whole-food sources like fish or poultry. If you're looking to improve your diet, you can also improve your sleep.

**Determine What Works Best For Your Situation**

Intermittent fasting, like any new habit, takes some time to become used to. It's okay to give oneself some leeway when it comes to scheduling. Alternatively, you may find that fasting for 8 hours is more manageable than fasting for 12 hours. In the end, it's all about what works best for you.

You may be able to sleep better if you eat at the same time each day. You should seek your doctor's advice before starting an intermittent fasting regimen, particularly if you are pregnant or have any medical problems.

## 2.5 Safety and Side Effects

Intermittent fasting's most common side effect is hunger.

Additionally, you may experience fatigue and a decrease in mental performance.

This may just be a short-term problem, as your body will need some time to adjust to the new eating plan.

Before attempting intermittent fasting, talk to your doctor if you have a health condition.

It's especially critical if you have the following conditions:

- Have issues with blood sugar regulation.

- Have low blood pressure.

- Are underweight.

- Take medications.

- Have diabetes.

- Have a history of eating disorders.

- Are a woman with a history of amenorrhea.

- Are a woman who is trying to get pregnant.

- Are breastfeeding or pregnant.

Intermittent fasting, on the other hand, has a very good safety record. If you're healthy and well-nourished, going without food for a while isn't risky.

# Chapter 3: The Medical Science Behind Intermittent Fasting

IF is an eating strategy that alternates between periods of fasting and eating. A growing body of evidence suggests that intermittent fasting may be an effective strategy for losing weight and preventing or even reversing various diseases. What's the secret? Is it safe to do so, as well?

In our evolutionary history, our bodies have developed the ability to go without nourishment for long periods. In prehistoric times, humans were hunter-gatherers who developed without food for lengthy periods and still flourished. Hunting games and gathering nuts and berries required a lot of time and effort.

Even 50 years ago, maintaining a healthy weight was a lot easier. It was an era when there were no television, no computers, and people stopped eating when the clock struck 11. This time the portions were smaller. As a result, "people were more active and engaged in physical activity."

Television, the internet, and other forms of media are readily available around the clock. Watching TV, playing video games, and chatting online keeps us up later and later into the night. For the majority of the day, we'll be sitting and snacking. "

Type 2 diabetes, Obesity, heart disease, and other ailments can result from a diet high in calories and low in physical activity. Intermittent fasting may be able to reverse these trends, according to scientific research.

There is also a scientific component to this, notably your body's ability to produce HGH. To understand why this is the case, I'd like to explain. The insulin our bodies make in response to food intake temporarily stores glucose in our bloodstreams for later use. Every day, we're assaulted with excessive sugar and fat content in our food because of the way we're raised. To put it another way, we're continually gaining weight because of this. Because food contains glucose, which is stored as fat, people gain weight. Our cells can use the glucose stored as energy when we practice intermittent fasting, which effectively reverses this process. Weight loss occurs when cells enter a condition of catabolism (decomposition). When we eat constantly, HGH production is reduced because our bodies absorb glucose from external sources, which inhibits HGH production. Human Growth Hormone (HGH) regulates metabolism, aids in muscle repair, and aids in fat loss. Up to a five-fold increase in HGH production can be achieved with intermittent fasting, according to research.

## 3.1 Is it Safe to Fast While Taking Medications?

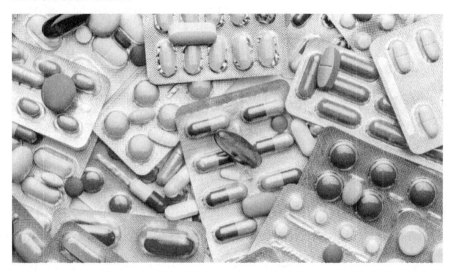

Discover how intermittent fasting may affect the side effects or absorption of any medications or supplements you're currently taking.

### Your Medication Regimen May Be Affected When You Fast

Your medicine and supplement regimen may be affected by fasting in numerous ways.

- Decrease or increase the effectiveness of your drugs or supplements by influencing their absorption.

- Some drugs and supplements can make their side effects worse if you fast. A common adverse effect is bloating and nausea, which can be avoided by eating a healthy diet.

## Supplements And Fasting

The first thing we need to discuss is your supplementation.

## Fat-Soluble Vitamins

Fat-soluble vitamins include vitamins D, A, E, and K. Taking them alongside a source of fat aids in their absorption more effectively. Vitamin D supplements are needed during the winter months, based on where you reside. Improvements in the immune system, mental well-being, physical vitality, and respiratory health have been demonstrated. Vitamin E is a fat-soluble vitamin that protects your cells from free radical damage by acting as an antioxidant. Supplements containing vitamin D should be taken during the eating window, with a meal high in healthy fats like olive oil, avocado, nuts and seeds, fish or red meat if you take vitamin D and an E-containing multivitamin.

## Iron Supplements

If you are taking iron pills, fasting may reduce your tolerance to any possible negative effects. Constipation and cramping are two common side effects of iron deficiency.

To make digestion easier, eat your iron supplements with food. Try a tbsp of mineral oil a day if iron causes constipation. Because the body does not absorb mineral oil, it aids in regularity.

Try varying the timing to see if you can find a winning combination. Iron absorption is inhibited by calcium, so make sure to eat iron with food that is not high in calcium. If you're taking an iron supplement, don't take it with milk or milk substitutes. If you're looking to get the most iron out of your food, citrus fruits are your biggest shot.

## Medications and Intermittent Fasting

### Diabetes Medications

Consult your doctor before embarking on an intermittent fasting regimen if you have diabetes or have difficulty controlling your blood sugar levels, especially if you use medication like Insulin or metformin. You may get diarrhea or flatulence if you take Metformin on an empty belly.

Hypoglycemia, a dangerously low blood sugar condition, can occur if you take diabetic medicine while on a fast. It's possible that hypoglycemia can activate your "fight or flight" reaction, resulting in weariness, dizziness, and a thumping heartbeat. Talk to your doctor about adjusting your prescription if your blood sugar levels continue to drop, as this could lead to seizures or a more serious condition.

### Thyroid Medication

Hypothyroidism, widely known as an underactive thyroid, can be treated with levothyroxine, a popular drug. It's a synthetic form of the thyroid hormone thyroxine, which is produced by the thyroid gland. This drug should only be used at specific times during the day. According to one study, thyroxine absorption is around 80% when people are fasting and drops to 60% after feeding. For the most part, medical professionals say that taking levothyroxine 30 to 1 hour before breakfast is the ideal timing. Levothyroxine on an empty belly before sleep enhanced thyroid hormone levels in a trial of 90 participants. What's the best piece of advice? Consult a doctor to determine the best time to take your medication. Regardless of the time of day, the goal is to maintain a consistent thyroid level throughout the week.

## Over-the-Counter Medications

It's that time of the month again, and do you ever go for aspirin to ease the pain? Ibuprofen or naproxen may be an option for you. All of these are NSAIDs available over-the-counter (Nonsteroidal anti-inflammatory drugs). Side effects such as heartburn and nausea can be reduced by taking NSAIDs with a meal or a cup of milk to help alleviate the discomfort. So, it is advisable to take over-the-counter medicines when you are eating. Always read the label and follow the directions on the bottle.

## Consuming Foods That May Interact with Medications

Certain nutrients may interact with certain medications in a harmful way.

There are several statins, which are drugs intended to decrease LDL-cholesterol, that interact with grapefruits. Because of their chemical, your body may have difficulty breaking down the statin, resulting in an elevated blood level and potentially dangerous side effects like rhabdomyolysis. It seems that only Lovastatin (Mevacor) and Simvastatin (Zocor) have this problem. If you consume a lot of grapefruit, it's usually not a problem. You should always consult with your pharmacist or doctor before taking any new medication or supplement.

Calcium channel blockers used to treat heart disease and high blood pressure can also be affected by the same mechanism of grapefruit's ability to increase blood levels of the drug. A rise in blood levels can exacerbate dizziness, constipation, and swelling of the lower limbs.

**Do Medication Interrupt Intermittent Fasting?**

Small levels of sugar can be found in gummy multivitamins. Breaking a fast is impossible if you consume sugar, which causes an insulin surge. The fat-soluble vitamins in gummy multivitamins can be better absorbed if they are taken with meals.

When taking medication, should you fast? It all depends on the situation. Maintain your specified medicine and supplement regimen. You should always consult with your pharmacist and doctor before taking any drug and double-check the directions on the bottle.

## 3.2 Can Intermittent Fasting Have a Negative Effect on Your Blood Pressure?

What is blood pressure in its simplest form? Let's review heart health and blood pressure quickly.

Blood pressure is a term that refers to the force exerted by the blood as it flows through your arteries. Arteries deliver oxygen and nutrients to your cells and aid in waste elimination. Hypertension, or high blood pressure, happens when the pressure of blood pumping through your arteries is constantly high, putting an undue strain on your heart to pump blood throughout your body!

It is estimated that 108 million people – have excessive blood pressure. According to the American Heart Association, hypertension is diagnosed when blood pressure measurements continuously exceed 130/80. For reference, a normal blood pressure reading is approximately 120/80.

Regrettably, high blood pressure can go unnoticed for years without symptoms, increasing your risk of stroke or heart attack. Consult your physician if you are concerned. During your annual checkups, they will almost certainly do regular screening tests.

## Blood Pressure and Fasting

Blood hypertension, cholesterol, and diabetes can all be lowered, and intermittent fasting can achieve weight loss. You can lower your risk of heart disease by addressing these four areas by fasting, as they are all risk factors. Fasting can cause an "electrolyte imbalance, raising your risk for heart arrhythmias," so always see your doctor before embarking on a fasting regimen.

It's no secret that fasting has been shown to reduce blood pressure. Blood pressure dropped in a study of 1425 persons who fasted for four to 21 days. The "rest and digest" state, also known as parasympathetic activity, lowers blood pressure while fasting. However, individuals only consumed 200-250 calories each day, which is barely enough for an ordinary adult to maintain their body weight. The results are encouraging, but they may not apply to the majority of people.

Nevertheless, a research of 32 people indicated that alternate-day fasting reduced blood pressure relative to non-fasters in the study group of participants. On their fasting day, they consumed 400-600 calories, while on the other days, they ate as they pleased.

Nutrition and Aging conducted a study of 25 individuals on a 16:8 fasting regimen in 2018 that found comparable outcomes in lowering blood pressure. Several studies have found a link between fasting and a reduction in blood pressure.

## Benefits Of Fasting For Your Cardiovascular System

Early findings on fasting are encouraging. While there may be a clear correlation between fasting and elevated blood pressure, there is no denying that fasting can be an effective way to improve one's health in general.

According to a meta-analysis of 13 trials, intermittent fasting is helpful for weight loss in healthy people with little effect on mood. LDL cholesterol, the "bad" cholesterol that raises the risk of atherosclerosis and heart disease, can also be reduced with this method. If you're concerned about diabetes, fasting may assist improve insulin sensitivity. All of these things work together to reduce your risk of cardiovascular disease!

## Is Intermittent Fasting Right For You?

Be aware that not everyone is a good candidate for an Intermittent fast. If you have any of the following conditions:

- Have a history of anorexia or bulimia

- Are pregnant

- Are over the age of 65

- Are you younger than 18 years old?

- Blood pressure has been low in the past.

Use prescribed medication. Consult with your physician beforehand.

Starting an Intermittent Fasting Program for Lower Blood Pressure: A Quick Start Guide

## Planned Meals

If you're fast, you may wind up eating less overall, so make the most of every bite. Remember that fasting only succeeds if you eat sensibly during the time you have set aside for eating. Making a weekly menu plan is a time-saving strategy.

## Increase Your Consumption Of Heart-Healthy Foods

Salmon, walnuts, olive oil, and avocado all include heart-healthy fats that lower your risk of heart disease. Make sure you eat at least one of these meals every day. You can lower your risk of heart disease, diabetes, and certain malignancies if you eat 30 grams or more of fiber each day. Whole grains like quinoa, oatmeal, lentils, kidney beans, chickpeas, fruit, seeds, nuts, and vegetables might help you get the most nutrients out of your eating window.

## Add Additional Minerals To Your Diet

Three minerals reduce blood pressure: magnesium, potassium, and calcium. How? You can lower your blood pressure by taking magnesium and potassium supplements. Potassium can also assist avoid heart arrhythmias if you're worried about them. Finally, calcium aids in the tightening and relaxing of your blood vessels as required.

- Focus on increasing your intake of these foods instead of taking supplements first. We have good news! Foods high in fiber and good fats also fall under this category.

- Pumpkin seeds, potatoes, cooked leafy greens, legumes, and whole grains are all good sources of magnesium.

- Bananas, cantaloupes, citrus fruits, apricots, sweet potatoes, prunes, and beets are all good sources of potassium.

Several dairy substitutes have calcium added, including low-fat or nonfat milk, sardines in their skins and bones, a variety of leafy greens and nuts, firm tofu, and white beans.

## Reduce The Amount Of Sodium In Your Diet

Please refrain from adding salt to the water. Your body relies on sodium, a mineral found in salt, to maintain a healthy balance of fluids. Consuming too much salt might cause your body to retain extra water, which can place additional strain on your cardiovascular system. You can lower your risk of heart disease-related death by cutting back on your sodium consumption. There is no need to eliminate salt and sodium from your diet if you don't feel like doing so. For fluid equilibrium, you do require a small amount of salt. Reduce your salt intake by cutting less on highly processed and pre-packaged foods.

Instead, eat more home-cooked meals prepared from nutritious ingredients. Look over the nutrition information for sauces and condiments. If a serving has more than 15% of the daily recommended amount of sodium, it's too much. Choose items with a salt content of no more than 15% of the DV, or even better, no more than 5% of the DV!

**If You're Expecting Or Nursing, Can You Safely Fast?**

Pregnant women should avoid fasting because they are consuming for the health of two individuals. Think about what your health needs to accomplish for the baby, not about losing weight. To ensure that you'll be able to breastfeed, you should eat a healthy diet now.

Keep in mind that the nutrients and food you feed your child are essential to their physical and mental development. Pregnant women may not have enough iron in their bodies. If you don't get all the iron you need in your diet, you run the risk of depriving your baby of the nutrients he or she needs. Your body provides your kid with the nutrients it needs, so you need to make sure you're getting enough of it yourself.

Fasting can negatively impact your baby's milk production and quality while nursing; therefore, it's better to avoid long periods of fasting if possible. Breastfeeding mothers should avoid fasting for more than 12-14 hours to avoid disrupting milk supply, despite the lack of medical or scientific evidence to the contrary. Stop fasting and eat more often throughout the day to see if that assists cure the problem if your milk supply is running low.

## 3.3 Why Intermittent Fasting Boosts Metabolism?

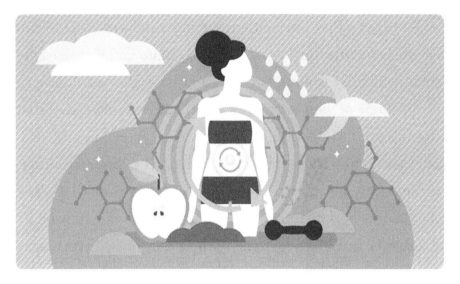

Fasting periods are followed by periods of regular eating, known as intermittent fasting (IF). Weight loss, disease prevention, and an extended life expectancy are all possible benefits of this diet. Some experts believe that it is a more effective method of weight loss than calorie restriction. If you skip meals, you may think that you're slowing your metabolic rate to preserve energy. Metabolism slows down when you go without eating for an extended amount of time.

Short-term fasting may increase rather than decrease your metabolism, as some older research has found. According to an older study, a three-day fast raised the metabolism of 11 healthy women by an astonishing 14%.

Compared to typical dieting, intermittent fasting appears to have the same or less detrimental effects on metabolism. Many people believe that intermittent fasting enhances metabolism because it reduces the loss of lean body mass and increases the rate at which fat is metabolized. To lose weight, you'll have to give up some of your lean body mass, but research shows that intermittent fasting results in a smaller percentage of lean body mass loss than regular dieting. The body's calorie-burning decreases if more lean body mass is preserved. On the other hand, short fasting periods cause the body to draw on its fat reserves and burn a higher proportion of its fat mass as energy.

# Chapter 4: How To Do Successful Intermittent Fasting?

## 4.1 Tricks To Make Intermittent Fasting Work

Intermittent fasting can help you get the most out of your Intermittent fasting experiences now that you have a better knowledge of what it is.

### Get into the Right Mindset

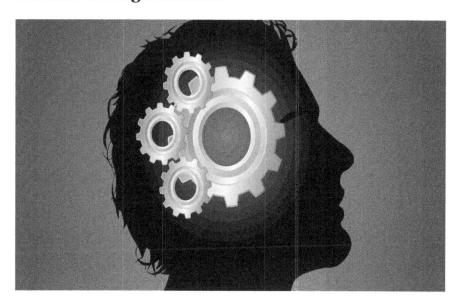

Many people fail at intermittent fasting because they lack the mental fortitude to succeed. Even before they see the desired results, they stop.

Intermittent fasting, or IF, should not be a one-time activity. You need to stick to it and make it a part of your daily routine.

You must also know what you want to achieve. Intermittent fasting is a popular method of weight loss. Having these goals in mind can help you determine whether or not IF is working for you.

If you stay with it, intermittent fasting can have a positive impact on your health. In addition to helping you lose weight, this eating plan can also improve your overall health and well-being. Fasting can lower blood pressure in obese people, according to a new study.

IF for Three to 24 weeks can help pre-diabetic patients control their blood sugar, glucose, and insulin levels, according to other studies. Fasting may also lessen the incidence of type 2 diabetes, heart disease, and non-alcoholic liver cancer. Memory and brain disorders may also be slowed by using this supplement. Even in animal experiments, short-term fasting has been shown to improve life expectancy.

Some persons, however, should not be considered IF candidates. Persons under 18, pregnant women, nursing mothers, people with weakened immune systems, and others with underlying medical disorders can all fall into this category.

Fasting should be avoided by people with a history of eating disorders since it can lead to a relapse of their disease if their eating habits are erratic or they go periods without eating.

If you're in good health, you should not begin an IF diet without consulting your doctor. Make sure you're in peak physical condition before you begin.

**Avoid Overeating**

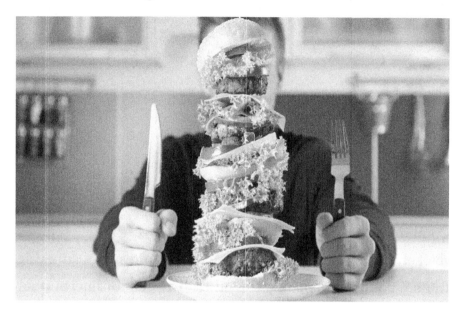

You'll need a strategy to avoid overeating during intermittent fasting. Prepare a healthy fruit or vegetable-packed dinner ahead of time so that you can eat it as soon as your fast is over. When eating, take your time, chew your meal thoroughly, and drink enough water to help your digestion. To avoid overeating, follow these methods to help you get a sense of fullness.

## Cut Down On Sugar And Carbs

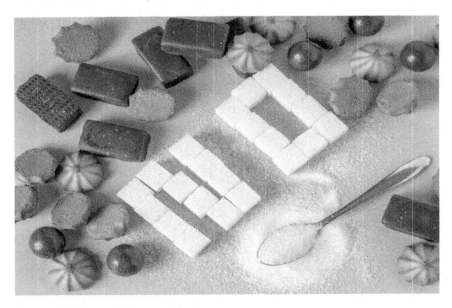

Combining intermittent fasting with a low-carb diet, such as the keto diet, is possible to lose weight. As a result of adhering to one, one is enriched by the other. The goal of intermittent fasting with a low-carbohydrate diet is to reduce blood sugar levels and burn fat by lowering carbohydrates (calories). Intermittent fasting and the low-carb keto diet are popular weight-loss and health-management strategies for many people.

The ketogenic diet is an outstanding example of low-carb, high-fat consumption, which begins by cutting your daily carb intake to between 20 and 50 grams, triggering a metabolic state known as ketosis. As a result of the metabolic process known as ketosis, your body must go from using glucose as its main energy source to burning fat as a primary energy source.

## Ketogenic Diet Intermittent Fasting

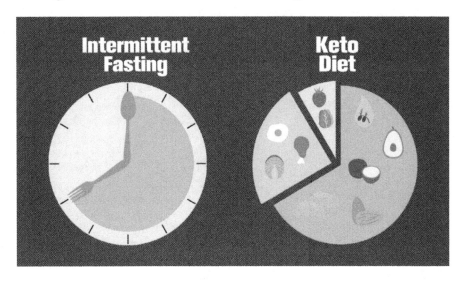

Intermittent fasting and the ketogenic diet may be generally safe. People with a history of disordered eating, such as pregnant women and breastfeeding, should avoid intermittent fasting. People with specific health issues should avoid intermittent fasting on the keto diet, including type 2 diabetes or heart disease.

However, it's crucial to remember that not everyone will benefit from combining the activities. Fasting on the keto diet may be too tough for some people, while others might have unpleasant effects, including overeating on non-fasting days, irritation, and tiredness.

Intermittent fasting isn't required to get into ketosis, although it can be a useful strategy. Anyone trying to lose weight and improve their health by reducing their carbohydrate intake can get by only following a well-balanced keto diet.

## Don't Tell Anyone Who Is Not Supportive

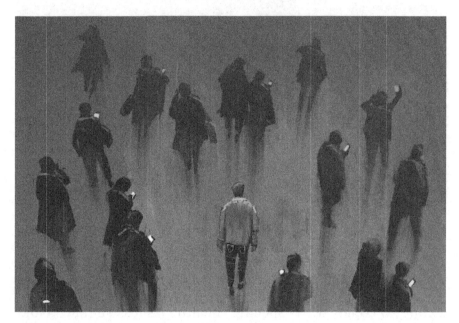

The desire for encouragement and support from others is natural, yet it is possible to accomplish your goals without them. Think about how many successful and remarkable people have taken the path less traveled. You have a lot of authority in your own right. You'll go a long way if you put your faith in that and don't give up.

## Opt For Satiating Meals

Anyone trying to lose weight should prioritize nutrient-dense foods such as fruits, whole grains, beans, vegetables, nuts, and seeds, as well as lean and dairy protein.

## Adapt Your Exercise Routine

If you enjoy working out on an empty belly, all the better! Continue to do what resonates for you. However, if you experience weakness or lightheadedness throughout your workout, it may be time to reassess your regimen.

## Keep track of The Journey

Keep track of your intermittent fasting journey by downloading the apps that best suit you.

## Start Listening To Your Body

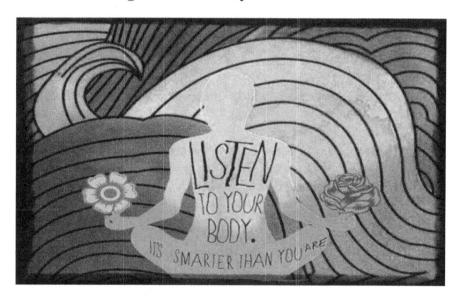

Intermittent fasting is a healthy and effective way to lose weight. There is no denying that it works for weight loss and overall health improvement, but it does not operate the same way for everyone. Bear in mind that each individual is unique.

Their health status, as well as their body's requirements, are all unique. What works for one person may not work for another. Therefore, listen to your body and do what feels right for you.

## 4.2 Tricks To Make Intermittent Fasting Easy

Adhering to an intermittent fasting diet can be difficult.

The following tips may assist individuals in staying on track and making intermittent fasting more manageable:

- Maintaining proper hydration. Throughout the day, drink plenty of water and calorie-free beverages, such as herbal teas.

- Avoiding food obsession. Plan several distractions for fasting days to keep your mind off food, such as trying to catch up on paperwork or watching a movie.

- Rest and relaxation. On fasting days, avoid vigorous activity, while gentle exercise like yoga may be good.

- Counting every calorie. If the chosen plan permits some calories throughout fasting times, choose nutrient-dense foods high in protein, fiber, and healthy fats. Beans, eggs, lentils, almonds, salmon, and avocado are all examples.

- Consuming foods in large quantities. Choose foods that are both full and low in calories, such as raw vegetables, popcorn, and fruits with high water content, such as melon and grapes.

- Increasing the flavor without increasing the calories. Garlic, spices, herbs, or vinegar should be used liberally to season foods. These foods are very low in calories yet packed with flavor, which may help alleviate hunger pangs.

- Following the fasting period with nutrient-dense foods. Consuming foods abundant in fiber, vitamins, minerals, other nutrients assists in maintaining stable blood sugar levels and preventing nutrient shortages. A healthy diet will also help you lose weight and improve your overall health.

## Benefits Of Intermittent Fasting

Numerous studies demonstrate that it can provide significant health and cognitive benefits. The following are some of the health advantages of intermittent fasting that are supported by evidence.

## Can Aid In Weight Loss And Visceral Fat Reduction

Many people who experiment with intermittent fasting do it to lose weight. In general, intermittent fasting causes you to eat fewer meals.

Unless you substitute by eating significantly more calories at other meals, you will consume fewer calories. Furthermore, intermittent fasting improves hormone function, which aids in weight loss.

Reduced insulin levels, increased HGH levels, and increased norepinephrine (noradrenaline) levels all contribute to the breakdown of body fat and its utilization for energy. As a result, fasting for a brief period raises your metabolic rate, allowing you to burn even more calories.

In other terms, intermittent fasting has a beneficial effect on both ends of the calorie spectrum. It improves your metabolic rate (burns more calories) and helps you eat less food (reduces calories).

## Changes The Way Cells, Hormones, And Genes Function

Fasting causes insulin levels to fall and human growth hormone (HGH) levels to rise. Additionally, your cells launch critical cellular repair processes and alter the expression of certain genes.

## Inflammation Reduction

Both intermittent fasting and overall calorie restriction have lower inflammatory levels, while clinical research is scarce. Oxidative stress is a precursor to aging and a variety of chronic diseases. It is caused by unstable chemicals known as free radicals. Free radicals interact with other critical molecules, such as DNA and protein, causing them to deteriorate.

Numerous studies indicate that intermittent fasting may strengthen the body's defenses against oxidative stress. Additionally, research indicates that intermittent fasting can aid in the battle against inflammation, another major factor in developing several common diseases.

## Loss of Weight

The majority of people begin IF to lose weight. And that assertion appears to be accurate, at least in the short run. According to a research, any variation of IF may help with weight loss. The researchers analyzed data from 13 trials and discovered that the average weight reduction for a two-week experiment varied from 1.3 percent to 8% for an 8-week trial.

That's good news if you're expecting to fast for losing weight, but the short duration of those trials leaves it unclear whether IF is durable and can help you keep excess weight off in the long run.

The other caveat is that the amount of weight loss appears to be comparable to that of another calorie-restricted plan, and based on how many calories you consume each day, you may even gain weight. After all, the diet does not prohibit the consumption of high-calorie items.

When done properly, intermittent fasting can be just as effective as traditional caloric restriction. Some people,

particularly those too busy to dedicate time to meal planning, may even consider a time-restricted diet simpler to follow than a keto or paleo diet.

**Cancer Cells**

Several studies have demonstrated that alternating-day fasting may lower cancer risk by reducing lymphoma growth, restricting tumor survival, and inhibiting cell spread. However, the studies that demonstrated the cancer benefit were all conducted on animals. Additional research is needed to validate the benefit in humans and understand the mechanism underlying these effects.

**Brain Benefits**

What is beneficial to the body is frequently beneficial to the brain as well. Intermittent fasting increases a variety of metabolic characteristics associated with brain function.

Intermittent fasting aids in the reduction of:

- excessive oxidative stress

- blood glucose levels

- inflammation

**Insulin Resistance**

Intermittent fasting has been proven in several studies in mice and rats to enhance the development of new nerve cells, which should have a beneficial effect on brain function.

Additionally, fasting increases the amount of a brain hormone called BDNF (brain-derived neurotrophic factor in the blood). A BDNF shortage has been linked to depression and a variety of other neurological disorders.

Additionally, animal studies have demonstrated that intermittent fasting defends the brain against stroke-related brain damage.

**Boost Energy Levels**

Apart from weight loss, another lesser-known advantage of intermittent fasting is an increase in energy. Consuming food multiple times daily requires our metabolism to cycle through cycles of carbohydrate breakdown and blood sugar conversion. It is eventually converted to energy or is retained in cells for later use. After the body consumes or stores glucose, the blood sugar level declines, affecting your strength and mental performance. This initiates a "hunger signal," which is likely to cause us to eat, and the process begins all over again. The continuous down and upcycle of blood sugar during the day strains our metabolism, resulting in decreased overall energy and mental function.

What is the difference between intermittent fasting and regular fasting? When fat is used for energy, it is slowly digested and must be processed (to ketones) in the liver before being used for energy. This process occurs gradually and regularly, without

peaks and valleys, which means we have more energy, feel better, and improve our focus and cognitive function.

**Renewal Of Cells**

Intermittent fasting enhances cellular regeneration. The newly formed cells and disease-fighting benefits act as brain boosters, assisting us in thinking more clearly, experiencing less depression and anxiety, and feeling happier than usual. With smart intermittent fasting techniques, we can even learn faster and sleep better. Yes, intermittent fasting can make you physically younger, psychologically healthier, and smarter than your years.

**Intermittent Fasting Muscle**

Almost all studies on intermittent fasting have been undertaken with the goal of weight loss. It is critical to understand that without activity, weight reduction will typically occur due to a reduction of both fat and lean muscle. Everything other than fat is considered lean mass, including muscle. This is true for both intermittent fasting and other types of diets.

As a result, several studies have revealed after many months of intermittent fasting, minor quantities of lean mass (1 kg or 2 lbs) may be lost. Other investigations, on the other hand, have revealed zero loss of lean mass.

Indeed, some experts feel that intermittent fasting may be more effective than non-fasting diets for preserving lean mass during weight loss, but additional research is needed on this topic. In general, intermittent fasting is unlikely to cause you to lose greater muscle mass than other weight loss programs.

## Longevity

One of the most intriguing aspects of intermittent fasting may be its capacity to prolong life. Intermittent fasting has been proven in mouse studies to extend longevity similarly to continuous calorie restriction.

Additionally, intermittent fasting has been demonstrated to prolong the lives of fruit flies. The results of several of these investigations were fairly spectacular. In a previous study, rats fasting every other day lived an average of 83 percent longer than rats that did not fast.

In a 2017 study, mice that were fasted every day observed an increase in lifespan of almost 13%. Daily fasting was also demonstrated to benefit male mice's overall health. It aided in delaying the onset of hepatocellular cancer and fatty liver disease, both prevalent in aging rats.

Although this has not been established in humans, intermittent fasting has become extremely fashionable among anti-aging enthusiasts. Given the proven benefits of intermittent fasting on metabolism and various health indicators, it is obvious that it could help you live a longer, healthier life.

## 4.3 Mindset For Successful Intermittent Fasting

Intermittent fasting is not a temporary weight loss technique! With intermittent fasting, you can give your body a well-deserved rest.

**Right Mindset**

Many people fail to reach their intermittent fasting goals because they lack the proper mindset. They resign before they even notice the desired changes.

Intermittent fasting, abbreviated as IF, should not be a one-time program. Indeed, you must be consistent and incorporate it into your lifestyle.

Additionally, you must be crystal clear about your objectives. Are you intermittent faster, for example, to lose weight?

These objectives will assist you in establishing benchmarks for determining whether or not IF is working for you.

For those who adhere to intermittent fasting, there are numerous health benefits. Not only is it an excellent diet plan for body fat loss since it helps you consume fewer calories, but it also has the potential to boost your overall wellness. According to research, fasting can aid in the reduction of blood pressure in obese individuals.

Other studies indicate that intermittent fasting for three to twenty-four weeks can aid in the regulation of blood sugar, glucose, and insulin levels in pre-diabetics. Additionally, fasting has decreased the risk of type 2 diabetes, some cardiac diseases, and non-alcoholic liver cancer. Additionally, it may help protect memory and reduce the progression of brain disorders. There is even evidence from animal research that repeated short-term fasting can increase lifespan.

However, not everyone should consider themselves candidates for IF. These persons may include children or those under 18, pregnant women, breastfeeding mothers, those with weakened immune systems, and those with other underlying medical issues.

Individuals who have an eating disorder or a history of eating disorders should also avoid fasting, as irregular eating habits and periods of not eating may trigger a recurrence of their disease. Even if you are in good health, you should not begin IF without first consulting your physician. Before you begin, you'll want to verify that you're in tip-top shape.

**The Mindset For Success**

Beginning your weight loss journey on a positive note is crucial for your overall success. Losing as soon as you start is one of the most disheartening things you can experience. But it's not uncommon for people to fail initially – breaking bad habits or forming new ones is hard for everyone.

Regarding health advantages, intermittent fasting (IF) has been connected to everything from boosting fat-burning to improving blood sugar balance to enhancing cardiovascular health. However, getting started might be a challenge. All of a sudden, you're subjecting your body to significant periods without food! Here are six ideas to help you get started with intermittent fasting successfully:

## Determinedness Is More Important Than Perfection

When embarking on a new endeavor, such as fasting, it's best to leave your ego at the door. Allow for the likelihood that your initial attempt will be deemed a failure. It is impossible to achieve perfection, so it is irrational to strive for it. To succeed at IF, you must have the encouraging and forgiving mentality of determination - the strength to pick yourself up and start again.

## Slowly Build Up Your Speed

The 16:8 technique does not necessitate a leap into the unknown. Begin with a 12-hour eating period and a 12-hour fasting period, like the 12:12 fast. Fasting at 8 pm and then fasting till 8 am the next morning is an example of a 12:12 fast. At first, the weight-maintenance outcomes of fasting at 12:12 versus 16:8 are identical, according to research. In the long run, lengthier fasting periods are more effective at improving blood pressure and insulin sensitivity. Once you've mastered the 12:12, you can gradually increase your fasting window.

**Drink A Lot Of Water**

Surely you've heard this advice on everything from skincare to mental wellness and weight loss. But if it weren't vital, it wouldn't be on the list. Don't forget to drink plenty of water every day (9 cups for women). It's possible to confuse hunger or boredom for hunger if you're thirsty. Drink a glass of water or a cup of hot tea first and see how you feel.

**Be Aware Of Your Cravings For A Snack**

Emotions can influence your eating habits, especially if you're a binge eater. Food can be a source of comfort in times of stress and mental illness. It's not uncommon for us to eat as a response to boredom. Focus on the purpose of your snacks, how quickly you consume them, and how attentive you are throughout your mealtimes when you are snacking. The key to breaking poor behaviors is to identify and address the fundamental cause of the problem. You should, of course, eat healthy snacks when you need a pick-me-up.

**I Can't Stop Thinking About Caffeine**

At the beginning of your journey with IF, you may experience a lack of energy. The good news is that caffeine-rich beverages like coffee and tea are acceptable on the IF diet. C caffeine can help you avoid weariness on a fast, and warm liquids can help you feel fuller.

Hold off on the whipped cream and confectioners' sugar, though. These are a certain way to end your fast, but they're also a waste of time and calories. If you're craving something sweet, consider monk fruit as an option. Zero-calorie sweeteners **are** made from plants that are less disruptive to blood sugar levels.

If you've heard whispers about bulletproof coffee and intermittent fasting, you're not the only one! You should know that MCT butter-coated coffee breaks your fast, even though that's a rabbit hole all its own. However, the fat in bulletproof coffee is the least disruptive to insulin of all macronutrients. Thus it isn't the most harmful. In addition, IF and ketosis can work together to maximize weight loss potential in numerous ways. But would the fat in your morning cup of joe sabotage your fast? Yes, in a nutshell.

## Maintaining A Healthy Lifestyle Is Essential To Overall Well-Being

You'll find it more difficult to stick to a diet like IF if your present habits are harmful. Good eating habits are much easier to maintain when you also pay attention to the rest of your lifestyle. A healthy diet and a healthy lifestyle are inseparable. For a healthy lifestyle, start by incorporating these practices into your daily routine:

The recommended amount of REM sleep for your age should be obtained:

- To achieve the best outcomes, go to bed early and get up early.

- Prioritize items that are both filling and invigorating when you're eating.

- Be sure to take your supplements on time.

## 4.4 Green Tea And Intermittent Fasting

Intermittent fasting doesn't mean you'll have to give up your beloved cup of green tea. Even if you're fasting, you're free to sip on a cup of green tea.

About 2 calories are contained in one cup of green tea. A few extra calories won't ruin your fast unless you're following an extremely rigorous regimen. On the contrary, drinking green tea during your fast would enable you to keep your fast for a longer period while also making it more bearable for you.

### Green Tea's Health Benefits When Consumed During A Fast

It may be sufficient to replace one glass of water with green tea while fasting. Fans of intermittent fasting will particularly appreciate the additional benefits of green tea.

Let's see if green tea can help you lose weight and stave off the effects of fasting fatigue.

## Weight Loss With Intermittent Fasting And Green Tea

Fasting on an intermittent basis has proven to be an effective weight-loss strategy for many people. Could drinking green tea help you lose weight?

To be honest, there isn't enough research to suggest that drinking green tea or any other beverage can help you lose weight. However, drinking green tea may help you lose weight in the long run, according to some research.

A cup of green tea can help curb one's appetite for many people. In addition to helping to suppress appetite, the caffeine in green tea has been shown to increase metabolic rate through a process known as thermogenesis.

The less hungry you are, the less inclined you are to break your fast, which is good news for those trying to lose weight while fasting. It's not just that your fasting intervals will be more joyful and less rife with hunger, either.

Green tea can also be a healthy alternative to sugary drinks and sodas when you're in the middle of a meal. Over a year, if you drink a cup of green tea instead of a can of soda, you'll save yourself thousands of calories.

### Intermittent fasting Fatigue and Green Tea

Fatigue is one of the most common negative effects of intermittent fasting for most people. This is a common cause of

breaking the fast, particularly for those new to intermittent fasting.

To overcome fasting tiredness, it's always preferable to address the underlying cause rather than simply masking the symptoms. In certain cases, all you need is a simple repair. As a result, caffeine can come in handy.

There are several benefits to green tea as an alternative to coffee for those who don't like the taste. Even though green tea has lower caffeine than coffee, it nevertheless has the same impact.

L-theanine, an amino acid found in green tea, acts with caffeine to enhance cognitive function while simultaneously reducing stress-related symptoms.

Instead of grabbing a cup of coffee when you're feeling lethargic after a fast, consider a cup of green tea. A cup of green tea should keep you awake without making you feel anxious or jittery, as is the case with coffee.

**Three Tips To Follow**

**Take A Sip Of Plain Green Tea Instead**

Number one on the list of requirements for a guilt-free fasting drink is that it contains zero calories (or as near as possible). No syrup, sugar or milk can ever be added to your drink while fasting.

Green tea can be enjoyed in its purest form — a cup of water and tea. If you've over-steeped the tea, you can put a slice of lemon to neutralize the bitterness, or you can use the natural zero-calorie sweetener stevia if you'd like some sweetness.

## Keep Green Tea Out Of The Way Of Bedtime

If you're looking to unwind with a soothing cup of tea before going to bed, avoid green tea. Green tea contains caffeine, which may disrupt your well-earned rest.

Try a caffeine-free form of green tea if you're still desiring green tea to satisfy your evening fasting appetite.

Teas with a relaxing effect are another fantastic alternative if you desire a warm fasting-friendly beverage before bed. Try chamomile, lavender, or teas labeled "bedtime," "sleep," or "night time" to help you relax and fall asleep.

## Choosing The Right Tea Is An Important Part Of The Process

Green tea shopping appears to be a simple process. Then again, there are some things to keep an eye out for.

Make sure there aren't any unwanted additives on the ingredients list before you buy the food. Additives such as honey and sugar are commonly used in iced teas, particularly green tea. Not a good choice for a fasting-safe beverage.

If you want to reap the most advantages from drinking green tea, aim for the most organic variety possible. Green tea in its most natural form is a loose-leaf or whole leaf. Both quality and taste are usually superior to those found in plastic containers. Organic products are the best option if you want to avoid the use of any chemicals.

## 4.5 Clean and Dirty Fasting

Fasting is either "clean" or "dirty," depending on how it is broken. When it comes to fasting, some experts recommend that you stick to water and nothing else, while others say that low-calorie beverages, MCT oil, stevia, and even a small amount of coffee creamer are OK.

With everything out of the way, let's get into the benefits, proof, pitfalls and takeaways of clean versus dry fasting.

### So, What Exactly Is A "Clean Fast?"

Water or non-caloric liquids such as tap water, black coffee, sparkling water, mineral waters, and black tea can all be consumed during a clean fast. It's very uncommon to come across material stating that clean fasting must be devoid of calories. However, a cup of black coffee has five calories. However, the amount of calories consumed is insignificant.

Only water and black coffee have no calories or sugars, although they include few nutrients. There aren't enough calories and

carbs to get your body out of fasting mode so it can keep using fat for energy instead of carbs.

## In A Clean Fasting Window, What Can You Eat And Drink?

Clean fasting necessitates that you stay hydrated. Drink plenty of water, whether it's sparkling, mineral, or distilled. Fruits, lemon slices, and herbs, on the other hand, should be avoided if you're on a clean fast. A "clean fast" is thwarted if you use these to flavor your water.

There is no insulin response to black coffee or tea; hence they are permitted on a clean fast. On the other hand, black coffee has been shown in certain studies to slightly raise insulin resistance.

Caffeine is a diuretic, which means it raises the amount of urine you produce. Coffee contains water, which negates the diuretic impact, so you shouldn't get dehydrated if you drink it in moderation. Coffee can be as hydrating as water, according to research. That, of course, is contingent upon your overall consumption. An increase in water lost through urination is possible if you consume more caffeine than 500 milligrams (approximately 4 cups of coffee).

For those worried about dehydration or insulin resistance, you may choose to stick with decaf black coffee or opt for naturally caffeine-free herbal teas like chamomile or hibiscus, which can

be consumed in small amounts during a clean fast. You don't need anything fancy; just some water will do!

**What Is The Purpose Of A "Dirty Fast"?**

You can practice dirty fasting during your fasting window by consuming only foods and beverages with fewer than 50 calories per serving. A little creamer in your coffee or a warm cup of bone broth makes your fasting a little less clean. Zero-calorie sweeteners can also be used to sweeten tea or soda.

**What Effects Do Artificial Sweeteners Have on Blood Sugar Levels?**

Low-calorie artificial sweeteners like aspartame are permitted in "dirty fasts." Although the word "artificial" may raise some red flags, even if you have diabetes, aspartame does not affect insulin levels or blood glucose homeostasis.

Sucralose and Splenda, both zero-calorie sweeteners, have also been shown to not cause an insulin response. However, this does not imply that artificial sweeteners are healthy. Artificial sweeteners such as aspartame and Splenda do not appear to have this impact, which is why they have become so popular as a replacement for table sugar.

Artificial sweeteners may or may not create problems, depending on the study, and there is no evidence that they are beneficial. Artificial sweeteners' effects on health will need to be studied over the long run.

**What Can You Consume During a Dirty Fasting Window?**

Here is a list of foods you can consume during a dirty fasting window. If you want to try dirty fasting, add them to beverages for flavor.

- 1 tbsp 2% cow's milk

- 1 tsp honey

- 2 tbsp almond milk

- 1 tbsp cream

- Sucralose/ Splenda and Stevia

- 1 tbsp maple syrup

- 1 tsp MCT oil

- 1 tbsp aspartame

- 1 cup bone broth

- Sugar-free chewing gum

- Water squeezed with the juice of 1 lemon

**Is Fasting Dirty a Factor in Your Weight Gain?**

There is little evidence to determine whether honey or cream is more effective at waking you up from a starved state. Cutting out MCT oil or bone broth may be necessary if you're not

experiencing the effects you'd hoped for. More studies comparing filthy and dry fasts are needed shortly.

However, your food patterns and food choices may be to blame for your inability to shed pounds. To gain a complete picture of your eating habits, pay close attention to what you're doing.

**Clean or Dirty Fasting: Which Is Better?**

Both methods of fasting are acceptable, depending on your goals. Ultimately, it's up to you to decide what feels right for you based on your preferences, progress, and goals. Combine the two methods, and don't be hesitant to do so!

Dirty fasts may provide you with the satisfaction and satiety you need to persevere in your fasting regime. For those who enjoy the taste of flavored water and coffee, there's nothing wrong with doing so! On the other hand, a clean fast can work if the taste is "negligible" and if you do not see the effects you want. It's up to you to see what works best for you!

## 4.6 Vegan Intermittent Fasting

With any diet or lifestyle, intermittent fasting can work. For weight loss, hormone imbalance, or preventing chronic disease, it is best to avoid eating high-calorie foods during intermittent fasting.

More than a diet, veganism is an attitude. As a lifestyle, veganism precludes all forms of animal abuse and exploitation.

Veganism has a positive impact on one's well-being. A vegan diet can help you lose weight and prevent the onset of chronic diseases.

### Intermittent Fasting As A Vegan Diet Has Numerous Advantages

Intermittent fasting and a vegetarian diet both have several health benefits, as everyone knows. These advantages can be enhanced by combining the two. According to numerous studies, a plant-based diet has been shown to have lower BMI than a meat-based diet. A vegan diet was proven to be more helpful in managing obesity and weight loss than a conventional diet.

According to the results of a recent study (RA), individuals with rheumatoid arthritis may benefit from vegetarianism and intermittent fasting. According to several experts, a vegan or plant-based diet dramatically lowers BMI, LDL cholesterol, total cholesterol, and blood glucose levels. Intermittent fasting with a strict vegan diet can help you lose weight and minimize your risk of developing chronic diseases.

**Who Can Take part in Vegan Intermittent Fasting?**

For those vegans who want to reduce weight and tone their bodies, intermittent vegan fasting is a terrific option.

Health risks associated with a vegan diet have been documented.

- caloric density is lowered
- , enhanced microbiome in the gut
- a greater ability to use insulin
- improved weight control

Nutritional deficits have been linked to plant-based diets, according to research. However, if they are well prepared, they can be suitable for all ages.

As a second benefit, intermittent fasting can increase growth hormone levels and improve performance training in the gym.

If you're trying to eat a healthy diet: Plant-based intermittent fasting necessitates that you schedule your meals accordingly. You'll be more aware of what you're putting in your body, which will lead to healthier eating habits.

**Who Shouldn't Try Vegan Intermittent Fasting?**

Dietary experimentation when pregnant or breastfeeding should be avoided at all costs, according to experts. Before embarking on a new diet, you should get the advice of your doctor.

For people with diabetes, fasting can cause fluctuations in blood sugar levels. You must have the proper supervision and your doctor's blessing to successfully practice intermittent vegan fasting while suffering from diabetes.

Suppose you have a medical condition that requires medication. Intermittent fasting is not advised if you have a background of any chronic illness or eating issue.

## 4.7 Myths About Fasting and Meal Frequency

I've compiled a list of 10 common misconceptions about intermittent fasting and meal frequency.

## 1. Consuming Food Frequently Increases Your Metabolism

As a general rule, many individuals assume that eating more frequently will help you burn more calories. Your body indeed burns calories when digesting food. What we call the "thermic effect of food" describes this (TEF).

TEF typically consumes 10% of your daily caloric intake. However, the most important metric is your daily caloric intake, not the frequency you gobble them down. If you want to lose weight, consuming three 1,001-calorie meals is better than six 500-calorie meals. If you have an average TEF of 11%, you will burn 300 calories in both circumstances.

As shown by numerous research, increasing or lowering the frequency of meals has little effect on the total number of calories burned.

## 2. You Gain Weight If You Don't Eat Your First Meal Of The Day.

A common misconception is that breakfast is essential to a healthy diet. Many people feel that skipping breakfast causes them to overheat, which leads to an increase in weight. When 283 overweight or obese adults were studied for 16 weeks, the subjects who had breakfast or not saw no variation in their weight.

On the other hand, breakfast does not have a significant impact on your weight, although there may be some variation among individuals. According to several studies, people who maintain their weight loss tend to eat breakfast regularly.

Furthermore, studies show that students who eat breakfast do better academically. Such consideration is critical in determining the best solution for you. Some people believe that eating breakfast is helpful, while others believe skipping it has no detrimental consequences.

## 3. You Can Lose Weight If You Eat Frequently

Eating more frequently does not affect weight loss because it does not increase your metabolism. A study of 16 obese adults revealed no difference in fat loss, weight, or hunger between those who ate three or six meals a day.

According to some people, eating can make it more difficult for them to stick to a healthy diet. Eat more frequently if you find it simpler to cut back on calories and junk food, but if you don't, that's fine too.

## 4. Hunger Can Be Lessened By Eating More Regularly

Some individuals believe that eating a few times a week will help alleviate hunger pangs and curb cravings. Mixed results might be found in regards to this.

However, some research has indicated that eating more frequently reduces hunger, while other studies have found no impact or even an increase. One study indicated that eating three high-protein meals a day reduced hunger more efficiently than eating six.

However, the individual's response may vary. It's usually a good thing to eat more frequently if it lessens your cravings. If you eat more frequently, you won't necessarily feel less hungry.

## 5. Fasting Induces Starvation In The Body

A common criticism of intermittent fasting is that it causes your body to go into famine mode, thereby stopping you from fat burning.

Weight loss can reduce the number of calories you burn over time, but this is true regardless of the weight loss approach you take.

Intermittent fasting does not appear to have a higher impact on calorie consumption than other weight loss methods.

Fasting For A Brief period Has The Potential To Raise Your Metabolic Rate.

Norepinephrine, a hormone that increases metabolism and tells fat cells to decompose body fat, is blamed. Fasting for up to 2 days has been shown to increase metabolism by 3.6–14%. You can reverse the results if you fast for too long and your metabolism slows down. Fasting each day for 23 days didn't lower metabolic rate, but it did result in an average fat mass loss of 4 percent, according to one study.

## 6. The Benefits Of Eating Frequently Outweigh The Drawbacks

Some people do believe that overeating is good for your health, while others disagree.

Autophagy, a cellular repair mechanism induced by fasting for a brief period, uses old and defective proteins as a source of energy. Anti-aging, cancer, and Alzheimer's disease protection may be provided by autophagy. There are numerous metabolic health benefits of occasional fasting.

According to some research, snacking or eating frequently may even be harmful to your health and increase your disease risk.

A high-calorie, frequent-meal diet, for example, was found to significantly increase liver fat, showing a greater risk of fatty liver disease. According to several observational studies, a higher incidence of colon cancer has been observed in persons who eat more often.

## 7. Fasting Intermittently Is Detrimental To Your Well-Being

Despite the misconceptions that it hurts your health, Intermittent fasting has been shown to provide several outstanding health benefits.

For example, it has been found to increase lifespan in animals when it comes to longevity and immunity. It also improves insulin sensitivity, inflammation, reduces oxidative stress and heart disease risk, and lowers blood pressure.

The hormone brain-derived neurotrophic factor (BDNF), which has been shown to protect against depression and other mental illnesses, may be increased as a side effect of the supplement.

## 8. Each Meal Provides Your Body With A Particular Amount Of Protein

According to some nutritionists, you should eat every two to three hours to get the most out of your workouts. Science, on the other hand, does not back this up.

Muscle mass is unaffected by increasing the frequency of your protein intake, according to research. Protein intake is far more significant than how many meals it's spread out over for most people.

## 9. You Need A Steady Supply Of Dietary Glucose For Your Brain

Some individuals believe that your brain will cease working if you don't eat carbs every few hours. Based on this idea, your brain is limited to glucose as a source of energy.

On the other hand, Gluconeogenesis is an easy way for your body to manufacture the glucose it needs. You can create ketone bodies from dietary fats even during long fasting, starvation, or extremely low-carb diets.

Glucose requirements in the brain can be considerably reduced by feeding the brain with ketone bodies. When they don't eat for some time, some people report feeling tired or jittery. Keep snacks on hand or eat more often if this is the case for you.

## 10. Overeating Is A Side Effect Of Intermittent Fasting

Intermittent fasting may lead to overeating during mealtimes, according to some people. While it is true that you may reflexively eat a little more after a fast to make up for calories lost, this compensation is not total. Those who fasted for 24 hours only ate an additional 500 calories the next day, significantly less than the 2,400 calories they had previously consumed.

Intermittent fasting helps you lose weight because it reduces your overall food intake and insulin levels while increasing norepinephrine levels, metabolism, and human growth hormone (HGH) levels.

Studies show that fasting for three to 24 weeks reduces belly fat and body weight on average by 3–8% and 4-7%, respectively. As a result, weight loss with intermittent fasting may be very effective.

## 4.8 Pros and Cons

While intermittent fasting can be an efficient method of losing weight and improving one's health, restricting one's eating to specified times of day may not be appropriate for everyone. Looking at the advantages and disadvantages will help you decide if it's worth giving it a shot.

**The Pros Of Intermittent Fasting**

**There Is No Calorie Counting**

Avoiding calorie tracking may be preferable to some persons who are striving for or maintaining a healthy weight. Either manually or through a smartphone app, keeping track of daily caloric intake and portion sizes can be time-consuming. Research released in 2011 indicated that pre-measured calorie-controlled foods increase the likelihood of people adhering to their diet regimens.

When it comes to calorie counting, intermittent fasting is a simple and effective solution. It is common for weight loss to occur due to calorie restriction when food is either eliminated or severely restricted at specific times of the day.

## The Instructions Are Straightforward

Many diets emphasize eating some foods while avoiding or restricting the consumption of others. It can take a long time to learn the ins and outs of a particular eating style. Intermittent fasting is a simple way to eat in accordance with the time of day or the day of the week. You only need a watch or a planner to know when to eat when you've chosen the ideal intermittent fasting method for you.

## No Restriction on Food

It's common knowledge that when you start a new diet, you start craving items you've been warned to avoid. A 2018 study found that an increased desire to eat is a crucial factor in the failure of weight loss efforts. 4

The problem is that this obstacle only applies to intermittent fasting plans. When you're not on a fasting schedule, you can eat anything you want during non-fasting times or days. These days are sometimes referred to as "feasting" days by researchers. Cutting back on unhealthy meals for a few days a week can help with weight loss, even if it's not the best approach to reap the benefits of intermittent fasting.

## It's Not Restricted By Macronutrients

Certain macronutrients are severely restricted in some popular diets. Many people, for example, follow a low-carb diet to improve their health or shed pounds. For weight loss or medical reasons, some people follow a low-fat diet.

Each of these programs necessitates a shift in eating habits, typically involving substituting familiar foods for unfamiliar ones. Cooking and grocery shopping may necessitate a new set of abilities. Intermittent fasting does not necessitate any of these skills. It's not possible to set a macronutrient target range, and no macronutrient is limited or prohibited.

## Weight Loss Is Encouraged

Those who engaged in clinical trials of intermittent fasting had a marked decline in fat mass, according to a 2018 assessment of the literature.

Intermittent fasting was also proven to be effective in lowering weight, regardless of one's BMI. According to the report, research on short-term weight loss has been done, but longer-term studies are needed.

Diets that limit calories on a routine basis may be just as beneficial as intermittent fasting. Intermittent fasting and traditional diets (continuous dietary restriction) had equivalent weight-loss advantages, according to a study published in 2018.

Scientists conducted a major meta-analysis in 2018 that included 11 studies that lasted between 7 and 24 weeks. Researchers found that intermittent fasting and constant energy restriction were equally effective when it came to metabolic improvement or weight loss. To conclude, more trials are required.

Weight-loss outcomes may also be affected by one's age. Intermittent fasting has been shown to have a positive effect on the health of both young and older men, according to a study published in Nutrition in 2018.

According to a new study, intermittent fasting reduced body mass in young men, but not in older men. However, both groups had the same amount of muscle power.

**Might Help People Live Longer**

Intermittent fasting has long been touted as a way to extend one's lifespan. When mice are put on calorie-restrictive diets, they appear to live longer and have lower incidences of various diseases, including malignancies, according to research from the National Institute on Aging.

Is this an advantage that extends to all living things? Those who advocate the diets say so. There is, however, no long-term research to back up this claim.

Religious fasting has been linked to long-term health advantages, according to a study released in 2011. Still, it was difficult to identify whether or not fasting was responsible for the positive results or if other factors were involved.

## Controlling Glucose

This eating approach may assist persons with type 2 diabetes in regulating their sugar levels through losing weight in overweight or obese people—but it could also worsen insulin sensitivity in others.

When fasting under nutritional guidance and medical supervision, a study published in 2018 found that insulin resistance could be reversed over seven months while blood sugars were kept under check. People with type 2 diabetes could quit using insulin medication, lose weight and reduce their waist circumference, and see an overall improvement in their blood glucose levels.

On the other hand, a bigger sample size in a 2019 study demonstrated a less significant influence on blood glucose control. Study participants with type 2 diabetes were followed up for 24 months to see if intermittent fasting or continuous calorie restriction improved their health. Both groups had an increase in HbA1c values.

Other studies have shown that blood glucose levels in patients with type 2 diabetes tend to rise over time despite a wide range of dietary changes.

## Cons Of Intermittent Fasting

### A Decrease In Physical Exertion

Intermittent fasting may result in a decrease in physical activity. Physical activity is not a part of most intermittent fasting programs, which is a shame.

It's hardly surprising that many who follow the programs may find themselves exhausted and unable to fulfill their daily step goals. Intermittent fasting has been presented as a way to study how it affects physical activity.

### Adverse Effects

In addition to the health benefits of intermittent fasting, research has found that the fasting phase of the eating plan can have some negative side effects. To name a few of the most prevalent side effects: moodiness, exhaustion, constipation, dehydration, poor sleep quality, and anemia.

You should avoid intermittent fasting if you have hypertension, high LDL cholesterol and uric acid levels in the blood and are at risk for cardiovascular disease, hyperglycemia, and liver and kidney disease.

### Medications

Certain negative effects can be alleviated if a patient takes their medication with food. Some medications, in fact, specifically advise that they be taken with a meal. As a result, it may be difficult to take medication when fasting.

Before embarking on an IF diet, anyone taking medication should consult their doctor to ensure that the fasting stage does not interfere with the medicine's efficacy or side effects.

## Intense Hunger

Those embarking on intermittent fasting (IF) diet are likely to suffer from intense hunger during the fasting phase. When they are around people who are eating normal meals and snacks, this hunger may get worse.

## Overeating

While in "feasting" mode, several protocols allow for unlimited meal quantity and frequency. Instead, customers can eat as much as they want, whenever they want.

Sadly, this can lead to people overeating. On days when "feasting" is permitted, you may feel compelled to overeat (or consume meals heavy in sodium, calories, fat, or added sugar) if you feel deprived following a day of complete fasting.

## There Is Little Emphasis On Eating Nutritious

Instead of focusing on food selection, the majority of people who practice intermittent fasting focus on timing. As a result, no foods (including those lacking in nutritional value) are discouraged, and no nutritionally beneficial foods are advocated. As a result, folks who follow the diet may not learn how to eat a healthy, balanced food.

It is unlikely that you will learn how to cook with healthy oils, eat more veggies, or pick whole grains over refined grains if you are on an intermittent fasting program for a short period.

## Limitations for the Long Term

Even while intermittent fasting is not a new concept, only a small number of studies have examined the potential health benefits of this eating pattern. As a result, it's difficult to say if the advantages will last. According to academics, long-term studies need to be done to verify if the eating plan is really safe for use beyond a few months.

For the time being, working with your healthcare professional to select and begin an IF program is the best course of action. Your healthcare practitioner can keep track of your progress, as well as any benefits or concerns you have, to make sure the diet you've chosen is right for you.

# Chapter 5: Mistakes

## 5.1  7 Deadly Mistakes to Avoid When Intermittent Fasting

### When You End a Fast, You Overeat.

After completing your first fast, you'll feel like a rock star. Even if you feel proud of yourself, that doesn't give you the license to abuse your good fortune. After a fast, you're likely to be hungry. Your post-fast calorie intake, however, may not compensate for the calories you dropped during your fast. If you feel this way, you may be able to excuse overeating and disregard all of your hard work.

Intermittent fasting can lower your insulin levels and encourage your body to use other energy sources to burn fat. When you eat too much after a fast, your insulin levels and blood sugar jump, which can cause a headache, nausea, and jitteriness. This can derail your fast and destroy your effort.

**Tips for Success:** You'll need a strategy to avoid overeating during intermittent fasting. Prepare a healthy fruit or vegetable-packed dinner ahead of time so that you can eat it as soon as your fast is over. When eating, take your time, chew your meal thoroughly, and drink enough water to help your digestion. To avoid overeating, follow these methods to help you get a sense of fullness.

### When You Make the Wrong Choice in Fasting.

Involves eating all of your day's nutrition in a specified period and not eating again for the rest of the day. If you're new to intermittent fasting, you may find this meal allotment a little strange at first. Irregular meal replacements are numerous intermittent fasting protocols that you can choose from when you're fasting.

Many people make the most common mistake in intermittent fasting (IF) by picking a fast that is too challenging or simply the improper fasting regimen for them. Think about it this way: if your body is used to eating every two hours, a 24-hour fast is likely to deplete your energy and make you feel down and depressed. Since most of us are awake well into the wee hours of the morning, it's a good idea not to start your fast at 5 pm. If you begin your fast early in the evening, you may find yourself unable to go to sleep until well into the next morning.

**Tips for Success:** To identify the best intermittent fasting method for you, do some study. You should select a fasting plan that is compatible with your current schedule and does not go too far in restricting your food intake. 14:10 will be a good starting point if you're a novice, as it requires you to fast for 14 hours and schedule all of your meals for the next 10 hours.

## During Your Feasting Window, You Eat Foods That Are Unhealthy For You

Another typical intermittent fasting blunder is overeating or consuming harmful items pre or post your fast. The items you eat after or before a fast are what will fuel your next fast, even though your body receives the maximum benefit when it has fasted. You won't reap the maximum benefits of a fast if you eat things that raise your blood sugar or make you feel full for a short time. What you consume when you're not fasting is the most important factor in how successful your fast will be.

**Tips for Success:** For your fast, your feasting window gives you the fuel you need. In this regard, stock up on complex carbs such as whole grains (like quinoa), veggies (like kale), and fruits (like bananas) for energy and fiber. Sugars, carbs and processed foods should be avoided. These simple carbs generate a spike in blood sugar and a surge in insulin, which your body will use as fuel instead of metabolizing fat rather than using fat as fuel. The appropriate nutrition guide can achieve maintaining energy, feeling less hungry, and losing more weight over time.

## Before Beginning A Fast, You Don't Eat Enough

During your "feasting window," you're supposed to eat everything you can and satiate your hunger before going on a fast. Ghrelin, the hunger hormone, tells your brain to eat when you're hungry. When you restrict your meal intake, your ghrelin

levels rise, and your hunger becomes more intense. During a fast, high levels of this hormone can cause you to feel hungry and exhausted.

**Tips for Success:** It's a common misconception that if you skip meals the day before your fast, you won't be able to fulfill your body's ghrelin hormone and would feel ravenous the entire time you're fasting. Fasting can't be healthy if you don't have a good time while doing it. As a result, it is important to eat a wide variety of healthful foods during your feasting period, including leafy greens, vegetables, fruits, and lean protein.

### You Lead An Unhealthy Lifestyle

Whether or not you are successful in losing weight is directly related to how you live your life. When it comes to losing weight, everything from your diet to how much sleep you receive impacts. The same can be said for lack of physical activity while on a fast. If you want to gain muscle and sculpt your ideal figure, you'll need to incorporate intermittent fasting, exercise, and a healthy lifestyle into your routine.

**Tips for Success:** There is no such thing as "intermittent fasting" or "intermittent fasting diet." Make it a priority to eat healthily, stay hydrated, and get a maximum of 8 hours of sleep every night. Intermittent fasting can increase fat burning by up to 20% when combined with exercise, so make an effort to stay active and get in three to five hours of exercise every week.

## You Aren't Getting Enough Water

Did you know that 70% of your body is made up of water? You need to drink a lot of water to stay hydrated with a water content this high. Not all of your daily water needs are met by the fluids you consume in the form of fluids you consume orally. 20% to 30% of your regular water intake comes from the food you eat, according to the USDA. To compensate for the water lost from your diet, you must drink more when fasting.

If you're following an intermittent fasting plan, it's a typical error to start your day with a cup of coffee or caffeinated tea. The moisture in your breath drained out nearly a liter of water from your body while you slept. As a diuretic, caffeine makes you more likely to urinate, which further depletes your body of water. Caffeine has been linked to increased insulin sensitivity, which makes you more likely to accumulate excess fat.

**Tips for Success:** Make sure you drink plenty of water. Before consuming any caffeinated beverages, make sure you drink a glass of water first thing in the morning. Drink 8 to 10 glasses of water each day, as well.

## When You Don't See Results Right Away, You Give Up

You're making a big mistake when you lose up on intermittent fasting because you don't see instant results. To lose weight and get rid of stubborn body fat, you'll have to put in a lot of effort over the long haul. After your first weight reduction, you should

expect to lose one to two pounds a week in water weight or bloat. According to research, there is a greater risk of weight gain if you shed your excess pounds too rapidly.

**Tips for Success:** Throughout your weight loss journey, embrace your body as it changes. You'll never notice overnight success with intermittent fasting, but it's a healthy and dynamic technique to permanently remove body fat.

When you're just getting started with an intermittent fasting regimen, you're bound to make some mistakes. It is possible to lose weight safely and effectively through intermittent fasting if you learn from the mistakes of others and adopt these beneficial guidelines into your lifestyle.

## 5.2 What Is A Fixed Mindset And What Is A Growth Mindset

For maximizing your human potential, having a positive mindset is arguably the most critical component.

The first step in determining which mentality is best for you is understanding the difference between a growth and a fixed mindset. The only way you can begin to alter your thinking and get the rewards that come with it is if you first comprehend and identify this issue.

There are many different types of fixed mindsets, but what exactly is one of them?

Fixed mindsets think that people are born with a specific level of intelligence or aptitude and can't do much about it. To these individuals, the effort is a sign of inadequacy, and they struggle to overcome obstacles.

**What Is A Growth Mindset?**

In a growth mindset, individuals believe that their intelligence and abilities may be improved upon through time. Rather than focusing on how smart they appear, these folks focus on how much effort it takes to succeed. These concepts are used to explain the underlying assumptions that people hold about learning, ability, and intelligence.

**Your Success Is Predicated on Your Mental Attitude**

People's success in life is influenced greatly by their mindset and the implications of trusting their ability. Personal development and happiness were found to be higher among those with a growth mentality.

Learning how to think in this way is a learned behavior based on how your parents taught you to believe in yourself, how your teachers influenced your behavior, and how you interpreted the outcomes you've been obtaining from your actions in the real world.

It is safe to assume that you are a person with a fixed mentality if you believe that you have already made up your mind. Even though you're currently in an unfavorable situation, having a

development mindset will help you achieve your goals regardless of your current circumstances.

**Your Growth Mindset Is Under Your Control**

The only constant in the world is changing, which is why the world is so unpredictable. We will certainly encounter naysayers and unexpected events, as well as encounter obstacles and pains. As long as you have a growth attitude, you can accept the situation and even benefit from it.

## 5.3 Your Mind As A Biggest Obstacle

Whatever you decide to do, your mind has a powerful hold on it. Pessimism or optimism can have a significant impact on the result of any endeavor. Perception is the term for this. The way you perceive events, people, and situations can significantly impact how you view them. Due to your preconceptions about the result of things, your thinking capacity might be used to sabotage your prospects of success. To make things easier on yourself, you may not have to put in as much effort.

The biggest roadblock in your way is you. I'll say it again: You are your own worst enemy! To achieve in life, you must use your mental power to transform any internal negative energy and, in turn, employ this force to increase your productivity.

### Take A Chance And Go With The Flow

Change is a part of life. It is the only consistent human activity. Therefore, you must practice adapting to change in your mental structure. Change is inevitable, and your success is determined by how well you can manipulate time and find new chances. To achieve this, your mind must be capable of easily adapting to change. To succeed, you must therefore organize your thoughts so that they can accommodate the constant flux of change.

## 5.4 Why Intermittent Fasting May Make You Gain Weight

### 1. You're Overindulging During Your Window to Lose Weight

What you consume is just as essential as when you eat, if not more important. The truth is that you can't expect to lose weight if you consume a lot of carbs and high-calorie, sugar-laden items. For the sake of your health, don't overeat since you know you won't be eating again for 16 hours.

In place of this, consume a healthy diet. You won't have any problems if you do that. Fresh fruits and vegetables, lean meats, seafood, and whole grains should be consumed. Isn't it wonderful? To lose weight, calculate your macros and consume a healthy diet.

Monitor your calorie intake as well. Put another way; you are probably overeating if you munch from when your window opens until shortly before your fasting window closes. As a general rule, you must cut calories to lose weight, but this must be done healthily.

## 2. You Are Not Consuming Sufficient Food During Your Window

Not eating enough can lead to problems, which may come as a shock to some people. How did that happen? If you don't eat enough during your eating window, you're more likely to overindulge in your next meal because you'll be so hungry. You'll feel so hungry that you may start eating and never stop.

In addition, the body keeps food in reserve as a defense mechanism. Rather than storing the extra pounds as lean muscle, your body will likely retain them as fat. You can still feed your body and lose weight at the same time if you calculate your macronutrients.

Reducing the fasting duration from 16 hours to 14 or 12 hours may help you avoid overeating during your feeding period if you are not eating while fasting. You can progressively increase the fasting period until you are back to 16 hours once everything is under control. Make a 20-hour fast your first attempt at a 24-hour fast to develop more control over your eating habits. Any of the fasting routines can be used to this principle. The most important thing is to eat regularly and do it in a way that supplies the body with the nutrients it needs.

## 3. Substitute More Protein In Your Diet

It can't be said enough: Protein is a crucial building component, whether it comes from vegan sources, protein powders, or foods like lean pork and poultry. A well-balanced diet rich in protein is essential for building and maintaining lean muscle mass. It's also healthy for your bones.

In addition to keeping you full, protein helps you get through the fasting window and into the eating window. A rise in insulin signals the body to begin storing fat when you eat sugary and processed foods. The hormone leptin, which alerts you when you are full, is also blocked by this surge. Fill up on delicious lean protein instead of carbs and refined sugar!

## 4. You Are Not Eating A Healthy Diet

When adopting an Intermittent Fasting routine, there are several reasons to consume a healthy diet:

- Trans fats and processed foods harm blood sugar levels.

- Intermittent Fasting improves insulin sensitivity and lowers blood sugar levels.

- Reduce your cravings and enhance your desire for healthful fruits and vegetables by avoiding refined sugar.

- Sweet potatoes, for example, are high in nutrients and low in the belly fat-storing properties of refined sugars.

- To maintain a healthy digestive system, it is important to eat foods that are rich in fiber.

- Reduce your energy drain by avoiding processed meals like muffins, fast food, sugary sports drinks, and false healthy foods such as instant oatmeal.

- Make sure to keep in mind that clean eating is not restricted in any way. It's still possible to eat a wide variety of delectable foods—and even dessert!

## 5.5   9   Mistakes   Beginners   Make   With Intermittent Fasting

In preparation for a weight reduction Intermittent Fasting experiment, you've stocked up on entire meals like chicken and fish, fruits and vegetables, and nutritious sides like legumes and quinoa. You're ready to get started. A major issue is that you haven't picked an IF plan that will help you succeed. If you are a regular, you may not want to fast for two of the six days you attend the gym each week.

Instead of rushing into a decision, take some time to think about your habits and schedule before making a decision.

## A Radical Start With Intermittent Fasting

A rash start is one of the most common blunders. If you don't ease into IF, you could be setting yourself up for failure. Eating inside a four-hour timeframe, as opposed to three regular-sized meals or six small meals, might be a difficult transition.

Instead, start slowly and build up your tolerance. The 16/8 technique recommends gradually extending the intervals between meals until you can operate effectively within 12 hours. A few minutes each day will bring you to the 8-hour window, so keep doing this until you do.

## You're Filling Your Stomach With the Wrong Foods

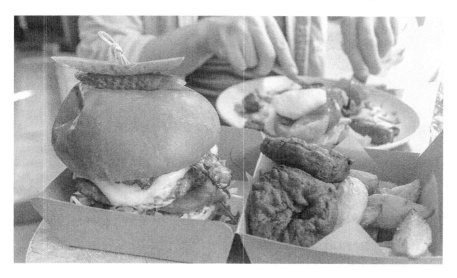

Overeating and eating the incorrect meals go hand-in-hand in Intermittent Fasting. You will not feel good if you eat fatty, refined, or sugary items during your 6-hour fasting window.

Eating Clean for Beginners explains how to eat nutritious, natural meals. Your diet should be centered around whole, unprocessed foods like nuts, legumes, grains, and vegetables and fruits high in protein and healthy fats. In addition, when you're not fasting, make sure you're following these guidelines:

**Instead Of Going Out To Eat, Eat At Home**

Get familiar with banned substances like high-fructose corn syrup and refined palm oil by reading nutrition labels

- Keep an eye out for sugars that aren't readily apparent, such as salt.

- Cook your food rather than relying on ready-to-eat meals.

- Make sure your meal is full of fiber, healthy fats and carbs, and lean proteins.

**Overconsumption In The Fasting Window**

One benefit of attempting Intermittent Fasting is that there is less time to eat, which results in a lower caloric intake. Some individuals may eat their normal daily caloric intake during the fasting period. As a result, your weight loss efforts may be in vain.

Don't eat your normal daily calorie intake of, say, 2000 in the window. Breaking the fast should be a time to eat between 1200 and 1500 calories per day instead. Fasting periods of 4, 6, or 8 hours will determine how many meals you eat. If you're in a state of deprivation and need to overeat, try rethinking your IF strategy or taking a day off to refocus and get back on track.

**Breaking The Intermittent Fast Without Knowing It**

There are a lot of fast breakers that you may not be aware of. Isn't it amazing how even the taste of sweets can cause your body to release insulin? Breaking a fast is made easier by the release of insulin as a result of this. Foods and supplements that can bring a fast to an end and produce an insulin response are listed here.

- Supplements containing maltodextrin and pectin as additions.

- Gummy bear vitamins, for example, are high in sugar and fat.

- Using xylitol-containing toothpaste and mouthwash

- Advil and other pain medicines may have sugar in the coating.

Don't make the mistake of breaking your Intermittent Fasting fast. When you're not eating, clean your teeth with a paste of baking soda and water, and be sure to read the instructions on vitamins and supplements before taking them.

## Calories Control In Your Fasting Window

Yes, it is possible to reduce your calorie intake. During your fasting period, you should not eat fewer than 1200 calories. As if that wasn't bad enough, it can also harm your metabolism. Slowing down your metabolism too much can cause you to lose muscle mass rather than gain weight.

The weekend is the best time to get your food prepped for the week ahead. You'll always have well-balanced, nutritious meals within reach. Healthy, nutritious and caloric-balanced meals are available when it's time to eat.

## Insufficient Water Intake While Fasting

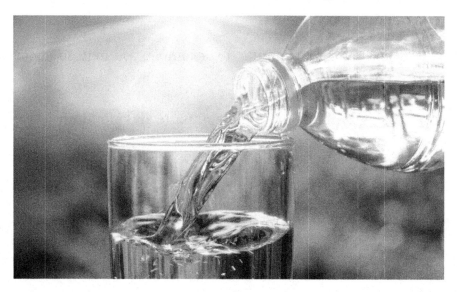

IF necessitates that you drink plenty of water. As a reminder, your body isn't taking in food-related fluids. Side effects might easily derail you if they are not taken care of. If you allow yourself to become dehydrated, muscle cramps, headaches, and hunger pangs might quickly arise.

Include the following in your daily routine to avoid this mistake and avoid unpleasant symptoms like headaches and cramping:

- Water

- Apple cider vinegar with water

- Black Coffee

- Herbal, oolong, black, or green tea

## 5.6 Being Excessively Critical Of Yourself If You Fail To Adhere To Intermittent Fasting

A single blunder does not equate to failure! There will be days when your IF regimen will be very difficult, and you will doubt your ability to complete it. If you feel the urge to take a break, go ahead and do so. A day of self-reflection will help you get back on track. Allow yourself occasional delights like a delicious protein smoothie or a hearty serving of beef and broccoli, and then get right back on track the next day.

Letting Intermittent Fasting encroach on every aspect of your life might be dangerous. Make it a part of your healthy routine, and don't forget to take care of yourself in other ways. Spend time reading, exercising, spending time with your family, and eating healthy. Becoming the best you can be is a full package.

## 5.7 Is Alcohol Consumption Allowed During Intermittent Fasting?

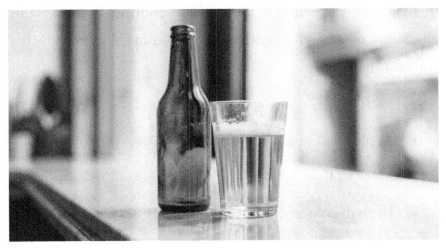

Even the tiniest quantity of calories can break your fast. As a result, you should not eat or drink anything that contains calories during fasting.

Drinking alcohol during a fasting period will break the fast because all alcoholic beverages contain calories. When you're fasting, it's best not to consume any alcohol at all.

To lose weight with intermittent fasting, you need to be in a calorie deficit at all times. For this reason, some people who practice intermittent fasting give themselves a maximum of 20 kcal per day throughout their fasting period.

Should you have a beer or a glass of wine? We strongly discourage it.

First and foremost, it is highly improbable that drinking alcohol will lengthen your fast. It doesn't fill you up and won't help you curb your appetite. Contrary to popular belief, most alcoholic beverages contain many carbohydrates, which raise insulin levels and make you feel even more hungry than before.

First of all, contrary to popular belief, alcoholic beverages contain a large number of calories. How many calories are in 20 ounces of booze?

- 2 tbsp. red wine

- 2/3 tbsp whiskey, vodka, rum, or gin

- 3 tbsp. beer

It doesn't seem worth it to break your fast for something like that, right? To keep hunger at bay, just add a tiny amount of cream to your morning cup of coffee or tea.

Having established that drinking alcohol during a fasting period would be counterproductive, let's check if it's possible to eat while on an intermittent fast.

## Is Alcohol Consumption Permitted During An Intermittent Fasting Eating Window?

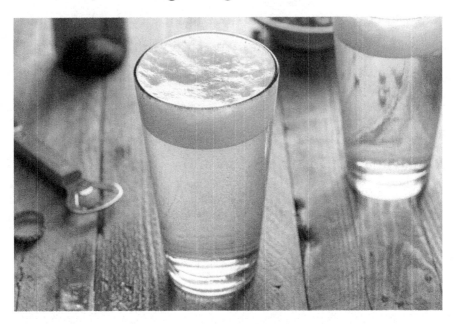

You don't have to limit yourself to a specific diet when you fast intermittently. When it comes to intermittent fasting, timing is everything. That means you can still have a glass of wine with dinner or a margarita on a night out while adhering to an intermittent fasting diet. The only requirement is that you must eat throughout this time.

Recall that intermittent fasting reduces your caloric intake. That's how it works! As a result, if you take the same number of calories while not fasting, you will not lose weight.

Intermittent fasting alone is not enough to achieve long-term weight loss; you must also analyze your diet. These foods would be lower in calories and less high-calorie junk food like fast food

and sugary beverages. These calorie-dense foods and beverages are devoid of essential nutrients like antioxidants, minerals, vitamins, and fiber.

Let's not overlook the fact that alcohol reduces your inhibitions when it comes to making eating decisions. When you drink alcohol, you are more likely to engage in impulsive nibbling and binge eating.

Avoid drinking alcohol while on an intermittent fasting diet if your primary goal is to shed pounds.

## 5.8 Exercise While Fasting

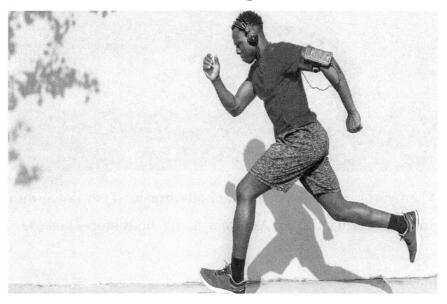

Exercise is permissible even for those who are fasting. Some people believe that working out while IF can be beneficial to their health. Among them:

**Autophagy**

Autophagy may be boosted by exercise and fasting, according to a review of studies.

The body's autophagy mechanism can destroy cells that are no longer needed or that have been damaged.

**Weight loss**

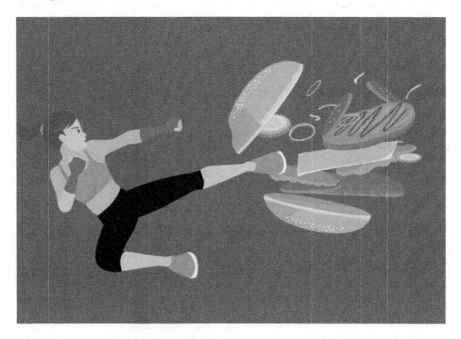

When carbs are consumed, the body breaks them down into glucose, a form of sugar. As glycogen, the body stores glucose.

Glycogen reserves are depleted during fasting, according to studies. This means that your body starts burning fat for energy when you exercise, which could aid in weight loss.

According to one study, people who exercised while fasted lost more fat than those who did so after a meal. The results of other investigations, on the other hand, have been somewhat different.

According to a study conducted in 2014, persons who exercised after fasting overnight lost no more weight than those who ate before working out. Another mouse study found that IF led to effective weight loss in mice, with or without exercise.

A person must consume fewer calories each day than they expend to lose weight. IF may aid with weight loss because it restricts the number of calories a person consumes. A study comparing an IF diet to a calorie-restricted diet without fasting periods found no significant differences in weight loss.

**Anti-aging**

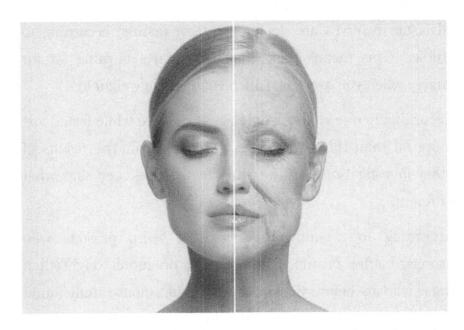

Researchers found that exercise and IF can reduce the aging process and the onset of diseases, according to research published in 2018. The reason for this is that exercise and IF may alter metabolism.

## 5.9 Not Exercising When Intermittent Fasting

Some people believe they cannot exercise during an IF period when this is the ideal situation. Exercise aids in the breakdown of stored fat. Additionally, exercise increases Human Growth Hormone, which aids in muscular growth. However, there are some guidelines to follow to get the most out of your workouts.

To maximize the effectiveness of your efforts, keep the following points in mind:

- Schedule workouts during eating periods and immediately follow with a nutritious carbohydrate and protein meal within thirty min of the exercise.

- If the workout is strenuous, ensure that you eat beforehand to replenish your glycogen stores.

- Adjust your exercise routine according to your fasting strategy; for example, if you fast for 24 hours, avoid planning an intense activity that day.

- Maintain adequate hydration during the fast, but especially during the workout.

- Pay attention to your body's signals; if you begin to feel faint or lightheaded, take a break or stop the workout.

## 5.10 Exercises You Can Do During Fasting

Intermittent fasting workouts should be done as soon as you wake up or as soon as possible afterward to compliment your body's natural circadian rhythm. To avoid disrupting sleep, it is best to avoid exercising (or eating) too soon to bedtime, as studies have shown that doing so can disrupt deep and REM sleep.

For the same hormonal reasons for exercising while fasting, it's best to avoid eating immediately following a workout. When you eat 2 to 3 hours after an exercise, growth hormone levels rise, which aids in fat loss and replenishes the energy you expended during the workout (sugar). Because of the stress of a high-intensity workout, hormones are shifted. After a noon workout, you can get the benefits of the hormone increase by not eating until 2 to 3 hours after that.

## Cardio

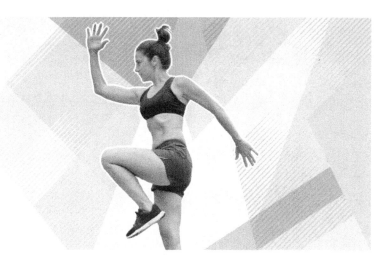

The hormonal benefits of fasted exercise are due to the decreased liver and muscle glycogen stores during fasting. At the same time, cardio is acceptable while on intermittent fasting; your performance will be determined by how adapted your body is to fat. If you're new to exercise and fasting, your performance may suffer slightly; it may take up to 6 months for some athletes to properly adapt to this new food source. For instance, if you are a competitive athlete whose primary goal is race performance, do not switch to fasting practice a couple of weeks before a contest.

If you're performing cardio in a fasted condition, avoid prolonging the fast post-workout and instead refuel afterward.

## Sprint Training

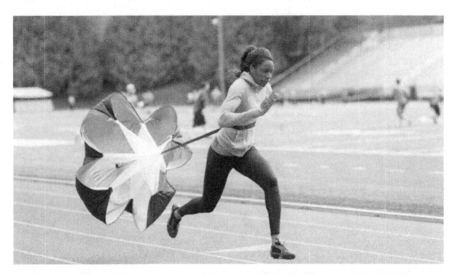

Sprint training consists of 15-30 minute intervals of vigorous activity followed by rest. Not only is it time-efficient, but research indicates that it gives health benefits not available through aerobic exercise alone, such as a significant increase in human growth hormone (HGH). Sprint training has numerous benefits, including enhanced muscular and brain strength and stamina, improved body composition, increased testosterone levels, increased growth hormone, improved brain function, and decreased depression. All of these benefits are enhanced when sprint training is combined with intermittent fasting. Sprint training is the optimal exercise style to add to your fasted time, and you can keep fasting 2 to 3 hours post-workout to maximize the advantages.

## Lifting Weights

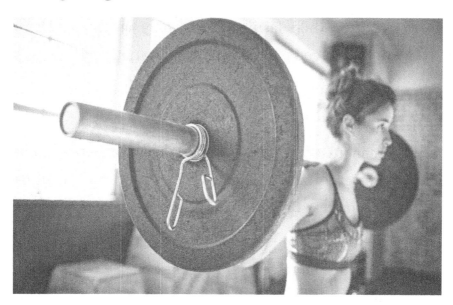

Weightlifting while fasting is also acceptable, but you must consider the significance of glucose in muscle regeneration following a strenuous weight-lifting workout, especially while fasting. When you exercise while fasting, your glycogen stores are reduced. If your day's workout includes heavy lifting, you can perform it while fasting, but you should prioritize eating a meal immediately afterward. Unlike a brief training session, heavy lifting places the body under stress that requires immediate refeed. As with exercise sessions, lifting weights while fasting may temporarily reduce your strength as your body becomes used to being a "fat burner." As a result, you may choose to schedule weight-lifting sessions after meals and combine fasted exercise on days when you undertake burst-style training.

**To summarize:**

- Workout while fasting is not only acceptable, it is extremely good for hormone optimization ;

- By combining intermittent fasting and burst training, you may maximize the benefits of both;

- The short-term effects of fasting on your performance in weight training and cardio can be mitigated by incorporating these activities into your daily routine.

- Early in the day is the optimum time to integrate exercise while fasting to fit the circadian rhythm of the body;

- You can also reap the benefits of fasting after your workout if you aren't partaking in heavyweight training or endurance cardio.

## What are the safest ways to work out when you're fasting?

When it comes to weight loss and exercise, long-term sustainability is critical. Maintaining your fitness level while doing IF is essential if you want to lose weight and lose body fat at the same time. That's why we've put together a list of helpful advice from the pros.

**Consume a meal shortly before engaging in a moderate- to high-intensity workout.**

Here's where knowing when to eat plays a role. Eat close to the end of a moderate or intense workout. Your body will be able to draw on glycogen stores during your workout.

**Drink plenty of water.**

Fasting does not imply a complete lack of water intake. While fasting, he advises that you consume extra water.

**Ensure that your electrolytes are maintained.**

Take coconut water as a low-calorie hydration source. 'It replaces electrolytes, is low calorie, and has a pleasant flavor. The sugar in sports drinks and Gatorade is considerable, so don't overdo it.

**Intensity and duration should be kept relatively modest.**

Take a rest if you begin to feel dizzy after exerting yourself too much. Pay attention to your body's signals.

Consider what kind of speed you'd like to go to.

Low-intensity workouts such as:

- walking
- relaxation through yoga
- light Pilates

The 16:8 fast, however, doesn't necessitate that you follow a specific fitness regimen during the 16-hour fasting window.

# Chapter 6: Frequently Asked Questions

Here is a collection of frequently asked questions concerning intermittent fasting.

- **When is it too much to fast?**

  Fasting for more than 24 hours can be challenging, and if you continue, you may experience discomfort. Even the 16 / 8 Method is considered tough by some. Always experiment with a variety of fasting methods to determine which one works best for your schedule and leaves you feeling the healthiest each day. The simplest technique to lose weight when fasting is to adhere to a specific protocol. IF can be implemented in a number of different ways.

  It's easy to see why the 16/8 diet is so popular; it restricts calories twice a week and is relatively straightforward to follow. However, alternative diets such as the 5/2 and alternate-day diets restrict calories just every other day. Because there has been insufficient study to determine if one method is superior than another, it is prudent to try a few different ones and determine which one works best for your lifestyle and physique.

- **Is Water Allowed During a Fast?**

Yes. Caffeinated liquids such as water, coffee, or tea are acceptable. Avoid sweetening your coffee. A modest amount of cream or milk is OK. Fasting is an excellent time to drink coffee because it can help stave off hunger.

- **How does intermittent fasting work scientifically?**

The diet is most effective when you abstain from eating at night. This includes no nibbles in between meals or before bedtime. Although this is not uniformly true, many people report success when they eat between 10 a.m. and 6 p.m.

- **Isn't skipping breakfast harmful for you?**

No. The issue is that the vast majority of persons categorised as breakfast skippers live unhealthy lives. Intermittent fasting is healthy as long as you consume a good food for the remainder of the day.

- **How difficult is it to adhere to this diet and how long does it take?**

At first, it may be difficult, but as your body adjusts to a new way of eating, the diet gets less onerous. The objective is to develop a more conscious awareness of what and when you eat. Apart from intermittent fasting, I advocate for regular physical activity, a sugar-free diet, and a concentration on whole foods such as fruits and vegetables, legumes, and grains.

- **May I take vitamins and other supplements while fasting?**

  Yes. Keep in mind that some supplements, especially fat-soluble vitamins, may perform better when taken with food.

- **What is the optimal time of day for fasting?**

  After approximately 12 hours of fasting, the body begins fat breakdown, which typically peaks between 16 and 24 hours.

- **Is Exercise Safe While Fasting?**

  Exercising while fasting is absolutely OK. Some people recommend ingesting branched chain amino acids before to a fasted workout (BCAAs).

- **How many fasting days per week are recommended?**

  On average, fasting can last up to 16 hours every day. The most popular method is to skip breakfast the following morning after having your last meal of the day the previous day. Another alternative is intermittent fasting, which involves fasting for 24 hours at a time, up to twice a week.

- **Can you lose muscle mass while fasting?**

  Muscle loss is a possibility with any weight loss method, which is why strength training and a high-protein diet are critical. Regular calorie restriction, according to one study, results in greater muscle loss than intermittent fasting.

- **How much food am I allowed to take during the eating period?**

  If you want to lose weight, you should aim for a weekly weight loss of one to one and a half to two pounds. To lose one pound per week, you should strive to cut 500 calories from your daily caloric intake.

- **Should I anticipate a slowed metabolism if I fast?**

  No. Short-term fasting has been demonstrated in some trials to improve metabolism. On the other side, longer fasts, such as those lasting three days or more, have the potential to slow metabolism.

- **Should certain beverages be avoided during the fasting period?**

  Water, water, and a little bit more water. If you intend to fast, you should consume enough of water. Additionally, broth derived from vegetables, poultry, or bones can be consumed. Avoid liquids with a high caffeine content, such as soda.

- **Is calorie counting a part of it?**

There is no guarantee, but your caloric intake will drop if you stop eating snacks before bed and go long periods without eating. You'll also be eating fewer calories because of the higher proportion of plant-based items in your diet.

- **Are Children Allowed to Fast?**

It's probably not a good idea to let your kid fast.

- **Does intermittent fasting pose a risk to certain medical conditions?**

Diabetics, people with a history of eating problems such as anorexia or bulimia, and pregnant or breastfeeding women should not undergo fasting unless they are under the strict supervision of a doctor or nurse practitioner.

- **Are there any additional advantages to intermittent fasting besides weight loss?**

Additional health benefits include lowering cholesterol, improving glucose control, and reducing liver fat while reducing blood pressure. People feel more energy, greater coordination, and better sleep as a result of fasting. Your body's natural circadian rhythm (eat during the day, sleep at night) promotes deep sleep. Fasting, which results in caloric restriction, has also been demonstrated to improve the longevity of even healthy individuals. Breast cancer recurrences may also be reduced by fasting, according to research.

- **For whom is intermittent fasting the most beneficial?**

Intermittent fasting isn't suitable for everyone. To help those who have struggled to shed pounds, this is a useful tool. A person's lifestyle and the decisions they make are the most important factors. What's going to work for them is a matter of weighing the possibilities.

# Conclusion

Fasting is a tool that should never be viewed as a rigorous diet. There are numerous factors to consider before beginning intermittent fasting, particularly for women. Women with eating problems, diabetes, or who are pregnant or nursing should avoid IF. If you do attempt it, begin gently and pay great attention to your satiety and hunger levels. If you are always hungry throughout the week or day, returning to a more normal meal routine may be preferable. Additionally, keep an eye out for symptoms such as weariness, mood changes, hunger, decreased energy, lack of concentration, and menstrual cycle disruption. Throughout the day, you should feel nourished, energized, and satisfied, not sleepy and hungry.

Intermittent fasting is a weight management technique that some people find effective. It is not suitable for everyone. If you choose to experiment with intermittent fasting, please remember that the quality of your food is critical. It is impossible to feast on ultra-processed foods during mealtimes and expect to lose weight or improve your health. You've undoubtedly engaged in a number of intermittent fasts over the course of your life.

If you've ever eaten dinner, slept late, and then skipped lunch the following day, you've already fasted for more than 16 hours. Certain individuals consume instinctively in this manner. In the morning, they just do not have an appetite.

Many people believe the 16/8 approach to intermittent fasting is the most basic and sustainable strategy; you may want to give it a try first. If you find the fast enjoyable and maintain a healthy state of mind throughout, you can graduate to more advanced fasts such as 24-hour fasts one to two times per week or eating 500 to 600 calories one to two days per week.

Another option is to fast whenever possible - simply skip meals when you are not hungry or lack the time to prepare them. It is not necessary to follow a structured intermittent fasting schedule to get some of the benefits.

Experiment with various methods until you discover one that appeals to you and fits your schedule. Additionally, you should consult with a healthcare professional prior to embarking on an intermittent fast.

# Intermittent Fasting For Women Over 50 Cookbook

*365-Days Healthy Recipes for Losing Weight with a 28-Days Diet Meal Plan*

By

**CAMILLE ROSE**

information herein is offered for informational purposes solely and is universal as so. The presentation of the information is without contract or any type of guarantee assurance. The trademarks that are used are without any consent, and the publication of the trademark is without permission or backing by the trademark owner. All trademarks and brands within this book are for clarifying purposes only and are owned by the owners themselves, not affiliated with this document.

# Contents

# Introduction

Intermittent fasting is an eating regimen in which you alternate between fasting and eating regularly. Intermittent fasting has been helping people lose weight and prevent or even reverse disease. Intermittent fasting entails going without food either completely or partially before eating normally again. According to several types of research, this type of eating can help you lose weight, improve your health, and live longer. Intermittent fasting advocates believe that it is simpler to stick to than typical calorie-controlled diets. Intermittent fasting is a personal experience for each person, and different approaches will suit different people.

The food we eat breaks down by enzymes in our gut, which becomes molecules in our circulation. Sugar and refined carbohydrates (think white flours and rice) are swiftly broken down into sugar, which our cells need for energy. If our cells don't use it all, it's stored as fat in our fat cells. On the other hand, sugar can only enter our cells through insulin, a hormone produced by the pancreas. Insulin is a hormone that transfers sugar and maintains it in fat cells.

If we don't snack between meals, our sugar levels will decline, and our fat cells will release their stored sugar to use as energy. If we allow our insulin levels to drop, we lose weight. The whole point of Intermittent Fasting is to allow sugar levels to drop low enough and long enough that fat is burned off.

Human studies comparing fasting every other day versus eating less every day found that both methods worked roughly equally well for weight loss, albeit fasting days were more difficult for people. As a result, it's quite fair to choose a low-calorie, plant-based Mediterranean diet. However, evidence shows that not all IF diets are created equal and that some IF diets can be effective and long-lasting, especially when accompanied by a nutritious plant-based diet.

We've evolved to follow the day/night cycle, often known as a circadian rhythm. Our metabolism has adapted to eating during the day and sleeping at night. Overeating at night has been linked to an increased risk of obesity and diabetes.

Researchers from the University of Alabama used this information to study a small group of obese males with pre-diabetes. They contrasted "early time-restricted feeding," a type of intermittent fasting in which all meals were squeezed into an early eight-hour period per day (7 am to 3 pm) or spread out over 12 hours a day (between 7 am and 7 pm). Both groups did not gain or lose weight. Still, the eight-hour group had much lower diabetic levels and significantly increased insulin sensitivity and significantly lower blood pressure after five weeks. What's the best part? The appetite of the eight-hour group was likewise dramatically reduced. They weren't hungry. Even people who didn't lose weight observed a significant increase in their metabolism merely by eating earlier in the day and extending the nocturnal fast. When you aren't eating, you can drink water or zero-calorie drinks like black coffee or tea.

Furthermore, "regular eating" during your period does not suggest that you are mad. You won't lose weight or become healthier if you stuff your face with high-calorie junk food, super-sized fried items, and desserts.

It's a fantastic way to reduce weight without resorting to fad diets or extremely calorie-restricting diets. You'll want to keep your calorie intake consistent when you initially start intermittent fasting. (Most people have larger meals in a shorter period.) Intermittent fasting is also an effective strategy to maintain muscle mass while losing weight.

Intermittent fasting is done in various methods, but it revolves around choosing regular eating and fasting times. You could, for example, only eat for eight hours a day and fast the rest of the time. You could also choose to eat only one meal per day, two times per week. You can choose from a range of intermittent fasting schedules.

There are seven ways to do intermitting fasting, 12 hours a day (Every day, a person must choose and follow a 12-hour fasting window), 16 hours a day (The 16:8 technique, often known as the Lean gains diet, involves fasting for 16 hours a day and then eating for 8 hours. Men fast for 16 hours a day and women fast for 14 hours on the 16:8 diet), fasting 2 days a week (The 5:2 diet requires people to eat an average amount of healthy food for five days and then cut their calorie consumption for the remaining two days. Men typically ingest 600 calories and women 500 calories during the two fasting days), alternate-day fasting (The alternate-day fasting strategy, which entails fasting every other day, has various versions. Some people practice alternate-day fasting by avoiding solid foods entirely on fasting days, while others allow up to 500 calories. People frequently opt to eat as much as they want on feeding days), weekly 24 hours fast (The Eat-Stop-Eat diet entails going without food for 24 hours at a time for one or two days a week. Many people fast from one meal to the next, or one meal to the next), meal skipping (Beginners may benefit from this flexible approach to intermittent fasting. It entails missing meals on occasion), and warrior diet. The Warrior Diet is quite intense. During a 20-hour fasting window, the Warrior Diet entails eating very little, usually just a few portions of raw fruit and vegetables, and then eating one massive meal at night. In most cases, the dining window is only 4 hours long.

# Chapter 1: Intermittent Fasting – The Basics

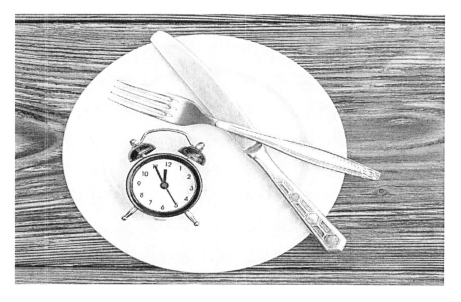

It's a method of planning your eats so that you get the most bang for your buck. Intermittent fasting does not alter you're eating habits; somewhat, it alters when you eat.

## 1.1 What is intermittent Fasting?

Intermittent fasting (IF) is a broad definition for any eating pattern that varies from not eating (fasting) with periods of eating. Various diet programs are available, including some that limit calories exclusively during particular hours during the day or specific periods of the week. The fundamental distinction between intermittent fasting and standard calorie-restriction regimens is that intermittent fasting does not restrict portions or foods, just when they are consumed.

One of the main reasons for women over 50 to pursue intermittent fasting is to get more incredible energy. Many women report a slight weight increase and worse sleep quality as they approach menopause. Both of these things might make you sleepy and sluggish. However, you may retrain your body to feel better by modifying when and how much you consume. If you're burning calories, intermittent fasting may let you consume what you want when you're hungry.

## 1.2 For How Many Hours Should a Woman Do Intermittent Fasting?

The 16/8 approach is the most prevalent approach for intermittent fasting. That implies you'll fast for 16 hours and then eat for 8 hours.

The 16 hours are usually completed when you are sleeping, therefore making it much more straightforward. This aids in hunger management and provides you with extra energy throughout the day. Intermittent fasting (IF), often known as time-restricted nutrition, entails skipping breakfast (TRF). Intermittent fasting is a food consumption strategy that alternates between fasting and eating at regular intervals.

## 1.3 Different Methods to Do Intermittent Fasting

Intermittent fasting may be accomplished in many ways. Continue reading to learn more about the many types of intermittent fasting.

- Fasting at least 12 hours a day.

- Fast for 16 hours a day.

- Fasting for twice a week.

- Alternate day fasting.

- A weekly 24- hours fast.

- The warrior diet.

- Meal Skipping.

**Fasting at least 12 hours a day**

The diet's guidelines are straightforward. Every day, a person must choose and follow a 12-hour fasting window.

According to some studies, fasting for 10–16 hours causes the body to convert fat storage into energy, releasing ketones into circulation. It should help you lose weight.

For novices, this form of intermittent fasting regimen may be a decent choice. Because the fasting interval is somewhat limited, most fasting happens when sleeping, and the individual may eat the same calories every day.

The most convenient approach to complete the 12-hour fast would be to include sleep time in the fasting period.

A person might, for example, fast between the hours of 7 p.m. and 7 a.m. They'd have to complete supper before 7 p.m. and wait until 7 a.m. to have breakfast, but they'd be sleeping for most of the time in between.

**Fast for 16 Hours a day**

The 16:8 technique often involves fasting for 16 hours a day and then eating for 8 hours. Women fast for 14 hours a day on the 16:8 diet. This intermittent fasting technique may be beneficial for those who have tried the 12-hour fast and found it ineffective.

People who fast this way complete their supper by 8 p.m., skip breakfast the following day and don't eat again until midday.

**Fasting for twice a week**

The 5:2 diet requires people to consume a standard quantity of healthy food for five days and then minimize their caloric intake for the remaining two days.

Women typically ingest 500 calories over their two fasting days.

Fasting days are typically extracted over the week. Between fasting days, there must be at least one non-fasting day. In a research of 107 overweight or fat women, it was shown that calorie restriction twice weekly and constant calorie counting both benefited weight reduction.

Twenty-three overweight ladies were studied to see how this fasting approach affected them. The ladies dropped 4.8 percent of their overall weight and 8.0 percent of their total body fat in one menstrual cycle. After 5 days of regular eating, the majority of the women's measures reverted to normal.

**Alternate Day Fasting**

The substitute day fasting strategy, which entails fasting every other day, has various versions.

Some individuals practice alternate-day fasting by avoiding solid meals entirely on fasting days, whereas others accept up to 500 calories. People often opt to eat as many as they want on feeding days.

According to one research, alternate-day fasting is good for weight reduction and heart health in both standard and fat individuals. Throughout 12 weeks, the 32 individuals dropped a mean of 5.2 kilograms (kg), or slightly over 11 pounds.

Alternate-day fasting is a more intense type of intermittent fasting that may not be appropriate for novices or people with specific medical issues. This form of fasting may also be hard to sustain over time.

**A weekly 24-hours Fast**

The Eat-Stop-Eat diet comprises skipping meals for 24 hours at a stretch for one or two days a week. Many individuals fast from one meal to the next or from one meal to the next.

During the fasting time, people on this diet plan may drink water, tea, and other calorie-free beverages.

On non-fasting days, people should resume their usual eating habits. This way of eating lowers a person's overall calorie consumption while leaving the individual's food choices unrestricted.

Fasting for 24 hours may be challenging, leading to weariness, headaches, and irritation. As the body reacts to this new way of eating, many individuals find that these symptoms become less severe over time.

Before attempting the 24-hour fast, people may benefit from doing a 12-hour or 16-hour fast.

**The Warrior Diet**

The Warrior Diet is something of intermittent fasting that is rather intense.

Throughout a 20-hour fasting timeframe, the Warrior Diet entails eating very little, generally only a few portions of organic fruit and vegetables, and then eating one huge meal at night. In most cases, the dining window is just 4 hours long.

This kind of intermittent fasting may be appropriate for persons who have previously tried other types of intermittent fasting. People should be sure to eat lots of veggies, proteins, and healthy fats throughout the 4-hour meal period. Carbohydrates should also be included.

**Meal Skipping**

Beginners may benefit from this radical approach to intermittent fasting. It entails missing meals on occasion. People may choose which meals to miss based on their hunger levels or time constraints. It is, nonetheless, essential to consume nutritious meals at each meal. Individuals who monitor and react to their bodies' snack cravings are more successful at meal skipping. People who promote intermittent fasting in this manner eat when they are starving and avoid foods when they are not. For some individuals, this may feel more comfortable than the other fasting strategies.

# 1.4 Benefits of Intermittent Fasting

Fasting has been demonstrated to have many advantages, including:

- o Reduces oxidative and inflammatory cell damage.

o Lowers blood sugar levels, decreasing the risk of diabetes or aiding in the management of diabetes if it has developed.

o Reduces abdominal fat and blood pressure, two major risk factors for heart disease.

o Enhances memory

o Multiple sclerosis and Parkinson's disease progression is slowed.

o Cancer risk is reduced.

o Assists with the healing of patients who have had surgery.

o Improved endurance as compared to calorie-restricted diets in general.

## 1.5 Maintaining Protein Intake

When you're fasting, it's critical to keep your protein consumption up.

Protein is required for the formation and repair of tissues such as bones, muscle, and cartilage, the production of enzymes and hormones and the maintenance of a healthy immune system. It also adds to the filling factor of meals. 45–60 grams of protein per day for vegetarians, doing this on 800 calories is more complicated. Therefore they may need to increase to roughly 900 calories per day to guarantee they receive enough.

Here are some essential calorie-counted tips to help you alter a dish, whether you're on an 800-calorie day or not, to improve nutritional profile or make a meal more satiating, whether you're on an 800-calorie day or not. They're convenient if you don't have time to make a whole meal and want to start with a plate of non-starchy vegetables or if you want to add something to a soup or salad.

## Meat and Seafood

- 75 grams chicken breast, cooked (115cals)

- 1 tablespoon chorizo chopped about 10 (29cals)

- 1 tablespoon about 7grams chopped fried bacon (23cals)

- 75g defrosted frozen cooked prawns (59cals)

- 45 grams tuna in oil, canned (85cals)

- 3 anchovies in oil, drained (17cals)

- Dairy and eggs are two types of foods that you may eat.

- 1 tablespoon grated cheese (about 10g) (41cals)

- 30g Cheddar – around the size of a matchbox (124cals)

- 30 grams halloumi, sliced, gently fried for 4–5 minutes in 1 tsp olive oil (145cals)

- 1 tablespoon full-fat live Greek yoghurt about 40 grams (37cals)

- 15 grams feta cheese (full fat) (54cals)

- 10 grams Parmesan cheese (42cals)

- 1 large egg (78cals)

## Vegetarian

- A handful of nuts about 10 grams, such as walnuts, almonds, or hazelnuts (185cals)

- 10 grams sesame seeds  (60cals)

- 15 grams of almonds (95cals)

- Tofu 100 grams (73cals)

- 80 grams edamame beans, cooked (85cals)

- 15 grams of mixed seeds (55cals)

- 100 grams lentils, cooked (143cals)

# Chapter 2: Breakfast Recipes

## 2.1 Pear and Cinnamon Porridge

A full and cozy breakfast. If you like, you may replace the pear with a shredded apple.

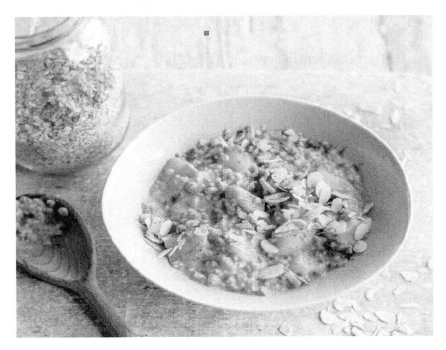

Preparation time: 5 minutes

Cooking time: 5-6 minutes

Serving: 1

**Ingredients**

- 30 gram jumbo porridge oats

- 1 Conference pear (around 135g) (peeled, cored and roughly chopped)

- ¼ teaspoon ground cinnamon

- 75ml full-fat milk

- 5 grams toasted flaked almonds (around 2 teaspoons)

## Instructions

In a small nonstick saucepan, combine the oats, pear, and cinnamon. Pour in the milk and 120ml water, and cook, stirring regularly, for 5–6 minutes, or until the oats are softened and creamy. To serve, pour into a deep bowl and top with flaked almonds.

## Nutritional facts

267 cals, Protein 7.5 g, Fats 8 g, Fiber 6 g, Carbs 38 g

---

# 2.2 Chocolate Granola

This simple meal is hearty and high in fiber, making it a great alternative to sugary cereals.

Preparation time: 5 minutes

Cooking time: 25 minutes

Serving: 8

## Ingredients

- 4 tablespoon coconut oil

- 1 tablespoon cocoa powder

- 1 tablespoon maple syrup

- 200 gram jumbo porridge oats

- 100 grams mixed nuts (roughly chopped)

- 75ml full-fat milk (per serving)

## Instructions

Preheat the oven to 170 degrees. In a large nonstick saucepan, mix the coconut oil, cocoa powder, and maple syrup over low heat, stirring frequently. Pullover the pan from the heat and mix in the oats till they are well coated. Bake for 15 minutes, spreading evenly across a baking surface. Take the pan out from oven and add the nuts. Return to the oven for 10 minutes more. Remove the tray from oven and allow it to cool and crisp up. Per person, serve 40g granola with 75ml milk.

## Nutritional facts

274 cals, Protein 8 g, Fats 16 g, Fiber 3 g, Carbs 22 g

## 2.3 Overnight Oats

The oats are softened by soaking them in milk overnight. The apple provides fiber and increases juiciness.

Preparation time: 12 hours

Cooking time: 0 minutes

Serving: 2

## Ingredients

- 1 small apple

- 60 grams jumbo porridge oats

- 25 grams toasted hazelnuts, roughly chopped

- 75 grams full-fat live Greek yogurt

- 100ml full-fat milk

- 1 tablespoon mixed seeds

- 50 grams blueberries or mixed berries

## Instructions

Grate the unpeeled apple coarsely, working your way around the fruit carefully and avoiding the core. In a mixing dish, combine the grated apple, oats, hazelnuts, yogurt, and milk. Refrigerate for several hours or overnight, covered. Serve with mixed seeds and berries on top.

## Nutritional facts

351 cals, Protein 10.5 g, Fats 20 g, Fiber 5.5 g, Carbs 30 g

# 2.4 Instant Porridge Cup

If you're on the go or have access to a kettle, this porridge is perfect. Non - fat milk powder is widely available in supermarkets and is often supplemented with vitamins.

Preparation time: 30 minutes

Cook time: 15 minutes

Serving 1

## Ingredients

- Porridge oats (40g)

- 1 tablespoon powdered dry skimmed milk

- 8 halves walnuts or pecans, coarsely chopped

## Instructions

To heat a cup, pour boiling water into it and then tilt it away. Pour quite enough heated water to cover the oats and dry, condensed powdered milk in the warmed cup — you'll need roughly 150ml.

Stir well and cover with a plate. Allow for 3–5 minutes of resting time. Check the consistency and, if necessary, add more water. Stir the oats one more to extract the starch and make them creamy. To serve, sprinkle the nuts on top.

## Nutritional facts

399 cals, Protein 12.5 g, Fats 24 g, Fiber 4.5 g, Carbs 31.5 g

---

## 2.5 Blueberry Pancakes

For the most outstanding results, use rolled porridge oats instead of the jumbo kind.

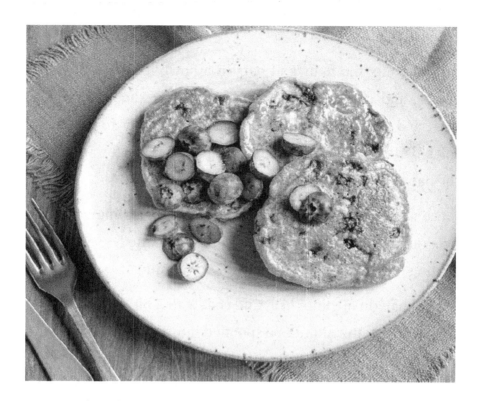

Preparation time: 20 minutes

Cook time: 10 minutes

Serving: 2

**Ingredients**

- 75 grams self-raising whole meal flour

- 15 grams oat porridge

- 1 large egg

- 100 milliliters of full-fat milk

- Blueberries ( 125grams )

- 2 tablespoons coconut oil

## Instructions

Add and mix the flour and oats in a bowl, form a well in the center, and crack the egg. Half of the milk should be added now, and everything should be whisked together to produce a thick batter. Add the remaining milk and mix vigorously until the batter is completely smooth.

Place the blueberries in a separate bowl, reserving some for decoration, and softly smash with the slotted spoon until putting to the batter and thoroughly combining.

Place a pan on medium heat and coat with a bit of the oil. One-sixth of the batter should be spooned into a messy heap on one side of the pan and gently spread. In the same manner, add two additional tablespoons. Sauté for 2 minutes, or until tiny bubbles emerge on the surface and the top begins to set, then gently turn and cook for 112–2 minutes on the second side. Cook the three remaining pancakes in the same method and transfer them to a hot plate. Serve with the blueberries that were set aside.

## Nutritional Facts

284 cals, Protein 12 g, Fats 9.5 g, Fiber 1.5 g, Carbs 37 g

## 2.6 Warm Berry with Yoghurt

A delectable mix that makes use of frozen fruit. If possible, use a fruit mix that contains sweet-tasting strawberries or cherries.

Preparation time: 10 minutes

Cooking time: 3-5 minutes

Serving: 2

**Ingredients**

- 100 grams frozen mixed berries (any kind)

- 2 dates, pitted and finely sliced

- 200 grams yogurt (full fat)

**Instructions**

In saucepan, sauté the frozen berries and dates over low heat for 3–5 minutes, or until the fruit has softened and warmed, stirring often. If necessary, add a few drops of water to help the fruit thaw. To serve, divide the yogurt into two dishes and top with the heated compote. Eat as soon as possible.

**Nutritional Facts**

190 cals, Protein 6 g, Fats, 10 g Fiber 2.5 g, Carbs 17 g

## 2.7 Turmeric Boost Breakfast

This spicy, creamy yogurt may be served as a breakfast or dessert. In either case, you'll benefit from turmeric's anti-inflammatory and cancer-fighting properties, which are amplified by the fat in the yogurt.

Preparation time: 15 minutes

Cook time: 20 minutes

Serving: 2

**Ingredients.**

- 1 peeled and sliced tiny banana (around 65 grams prepared weight).

- 150g live Greek yoghurt (full fat).

- 1/2–1 teaspoon turmeric powder (to taste).

- 1/4 teaspoon ginger powder

- 1/4 tsp cinnamon powder

- 8 halved pecans or walnuts, coarsely broken or chopped

**Instructions**

In a mixing basin, mash the banana coarsely with a fork. Sprinkle the turmeric, ginger, and cinnamon over the yogurt. Mix well, add a little touch of water if the yogurt is too dense to spread, then divide into two plates or glass tumblers, top with almonds, and serve.

**Nutritional Facts**

178cals, Protein 5.5 g, Fats 12.5 g, Fiber 1 g, Carbs 10.5 g

## 2.8 Banana and Pecan Muffin

A healthier replacement to a coffee shop muffin, this warm, fluffy morning delight is warm and fluffy. Serve with a sprinkling of fresh berries on top.

Preparation time: 10 minutes

Cooking time: 5 minutes

Serving: 2

## Ingredients

- 1 tablespoon coconut oil.

- 1 egg

- 1 small peeled ripe banana, minced with a fork

- 20 g almond flour

- 20g self-raising whole meal flour

- A quarter teaspoon of baking powder

- 8 halved pecans, coarsely chopped

- 12 teaspoon cinnamon powder

## Instructions

Lightly lubricate a microwave-safe mug with a bit of quantity of the oil.

Split the egg into the cup and beat it with a fork until it is completely smooth.

In a large mixing bowl, mix all the ingredients, including banana, almonds, flour, baking powder, pecans, cinnamon, and the remaining oil.

Microwave for approximately 112 minutes on high, or until risen and hard. The cake should have just started to shrink away from the mug's edges.

Allow for 1 minute of resting time before loosening the edges and tipping the muffin out of the cup. Serve it warm, cut in half.

**Nutritional Facts**

322 cals, Protein 10 g, Fast 25 g, Fiber 2.5 g, Carbs 14.5 g

## 2.9 Citrus Salad

This bright, light, and appealing breakfast may also be offered as a dessert. You may make the fruit the night before and keep it refrigerated in the fridge until you're ready to eat it, making it even more refreshing.

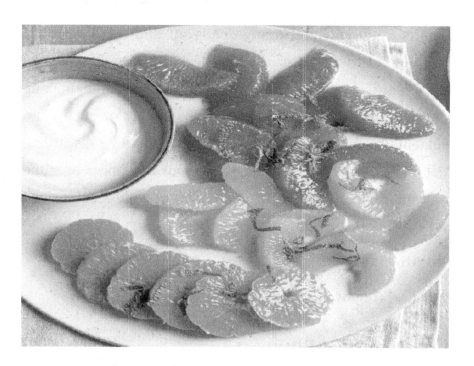

Preparation time: 5 minutes

Cooking time: 10 minutes

Servings: 2

## Ingredients

- 1 pink grapefruit

- 1 orange

- 1 clementine, tangerine or satsuma

- 4–5 fresh mint leaves, thinly sliced

- 100g Yoghurt

## Instructions

Cut the grapefruit and orange ends off and set them on a chopping board with a groove to collect any juice. Remove the skin and pith from both fruits with a tiny sharp knife, making your way around them. Slice the apple thinly or cut it into segments by turning it on its side. Pips should be discarded. Peel and finely slice the clementine. Pour any juices over the fruit and divide between two plates. Serve with Greek yogurt and a sprinkling of mint.

**Nutritional Facts**

135 cals, Protein 4.5 g, Fats 5.5 g, Fiber 3 g, Carbs 17 g

## 2.10 Breakfast Plums

Warm or cold, this dish is delicious. It might also be served as a light dessert.

Preparation time: 25 minutes

Cook time: 25 minutes

Serving: 2

**Ingredients**

- 4 plums (about 275g), stoned and halved
- 10–12 centimeter strips orange zest, peeled with a vegetable peeler
- 1 large orange
- 1/4 teaspoon ground cinnamon

- 100g Greek yogurt

- 15 g flaked almonds, roasted

**Instructions**

In a saucepan, place the plums. Combine the orange zest and juice, 150ml water, and the cinnamon in a mixing bowl. Lightly whisk the ingredients together. Take the liquid to a low boil, then cover with a lid and continue cooking for 10–15 minutes, or till the plums are softened but still maintain their form. Divide the plums into two dishes and top with Greek yogurt and toasted almonds to serve warm or cold.

**Nutritional Facts**

233 cals, Protein 6 g, Fats 9.5 g, Fiber 2.5 g, Carbs 30 g

## 2.11 Scrambled Eggs with Mushrooms and Spinach

Breakfast for one that is quick, low-calorie, and filling. Make sure you're using fresh eggs.

Preparation time: 20 minutes

Cooking time: 10 minutes

Servings: 1

**Ingredients**

- 2 medium eggs, chilled from the fridge

- 1 teaspoon olive oil or 5 gram butter

- 75g sliced tiny chestnut mushrooms
- Bunch of spinach Leaves

## Instructions

One Third, fill a pot halfway with water and pour to a low boil. Crack every egg into a bowl and gently pour one into the pan at a time. Cook for 3 minutes over a low flame, with the water barely boiling, until the egg whites are done, but the egg yolks are still runny. While the eggs are poaching, melt the butter or oil in a nonstick frying pan over medium heat and shallow fry the mushrooms for 2 to 3 minutes, or lightly browned. Toss the spinach with the mushrooms until it is slightly cooked. If you overcook it, a lot of liquid will come out. Add a sprinkle of sea salt and a generous dash of black pepper to taste. Place the mushrooms and spinach on a platter that has been warmed. Drain the eggs and lay them on top of the vegetables using a slotted spoon. To serve, season with a bit extra ground black pepper.

## Nutritional Facts

241 cals, Protein 21 g, Fats 17 g, Fiber 1 g, Carbs 0.5 g

## 2.12 Smoked Salmon Omelet

Lunch is both exquisite and speedy. The butter in the omelet adds more richness, but if you want, you may simply use olive oil. Serve with a mixed salad, and if dressed, add the additional calories.

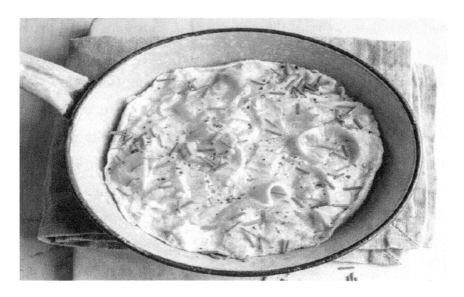

Preparation time: 10 minutes

Cooked time: 20 minutes

Servings: 1

**Ingredients**

- 2 eggs, big

- 1 tablespoon of butter

- 1 tablespoon extra-virgin olive oil

- 50g smoked salmon slices, thinly sliced

- Snipped fresh chives to serve

**Instructions**

In a mixing bowl, put the eggs and whisk them vigorously with a big whisk. Season with black pepper, ground. In a medium-size nonstick frying pan, melt the butter with the oil over moderate flame. Break the egg into the saucepan and wait a few seconds for it to fry. Draw the egg in from the edges of the pan towards the center using a wooden spoon, then allow the uncooked egg flow to fill the space. It should be done multiple times. The omelet will seem thicker and lighter as a result of this. Sprinkle the salmon strips on top and cook for a further 1–2 minutes, or until the omelet is gently browned beneath and set on top, and the salmon is warm and bright pink. If using, slide the omelet onto a dish, fold it, and top with freshly chopped chives.

**Nutritional Facts**

339 cals, Protein 30 g, Fats 24.5 g, Fiber 0 g, Carbs 0 g

## 2.13 Mushroom on Toasted Sourdough

A flavorful and simple supper that can easily be multiplied for additional servings. Cooking the mushrooms takes virtually as little time as toasting the bread.

Preparation time: 15 minutes

Cook time: 20 minutes

Serving: 1

**Ingredients**

- 1 tablespoon extra-virgin olive oil

- 2 big sliced Portobello mushrooms (140g)

- 1 sliver of wholegrain sourdough bread (about 20g)

- 12 peeled and smashed garlic cloves

- 14 teaspoon dried thyme or 2 teaspoon fresh thyme leaves

- 1 tablespoon balsamic vinaigrette

- A small bunch of finely chopped fresh parsley

- 2 thin slices of goat cheese (about 40g)

## Instructions

In a large size nonstick frying pan, heat the olive oil over high heat and cook the mushrooms, frequently tossing, for 3 minutes or lightly browned. Toast the bread in the meanwhile. Cook for 30 seconds, constantly stirring, after adding the garlic and herbs to the mushrooms. Toss in the vinegar and parsley for a few seconds. Stack the mushrooms on the bread, then top with goat's cheese and a good pinch of black pepper.

## Nutritional Facts

297cals, Protein 13 g, Fats 22 g, Fiber 1.5 g, Carbs 11 g

## 2.14 Sliced avocado on toast

This super-quick breakfast is a fantastic way to use up overripe avocados.

Preparation time: 10 minutes

Cook time: 10 minutes

Servings: 2

## Ingredients

- 2 slices wholegrain sourdough bread (about 20g).

- 25 grams walnut halves (about 10) 1 ripe medium avocado, stoned, skinned, and coarsely chopped.

- 1 deseeded and diced plump red chili or a teaspoon of crumbled dried chili flakes

- 2 tablespoon balsamic vinaigrette.

## Instructions

Roasted the bread and split it between two dishes (or served it all on one platter). In a small bowl, blend the avocado and walnuts with a fork. Splash the balsamic vinegar over the heated bread and sprinkle with the chili if used. To serve, season with sea salt and freshly ground black pepper.

## Nutritional Facts

289 cals, Protein 6 g, Fats 23.5 g, Fiber 5 g, Carbs 10.5 g

---

## 2.15 Baked Beans

One of the finest breakfasts is homemade baked beans. This easy variation is excellent for breakfast or as a side dish with grilled chicken or beef. It's also delicious, with crumbled cheese on top for a fast dinner.

Preparation time: 15 minutes

Cook times: 10 minutes

Serving: 2

## Ingredients

- 1 tablespoon extra-virgin olive oil

- 1 small peeled and coarsely chopped onion

- 1 peeled and smashed garlic clove

- 1 teaspoon smoked paprika, spicy or sweet to taste

- 400 g drained haricot beans

- 350 g tomato puree

- 1 tablespoon Worcestershire sauce (optional)

- 2 slices wholegrain bread, thinly sliced (each around 20g)

## Instructions

In a nonstick saucepan, heat the oil, add the onion, and gently cook for 3 to 4 minutes. Or till the potatoes are tender. Sauté for a few seconds longer, frequently stirring, after adding the garlic and paprika. Add the pureed tomatoes and Worcestershire sauce to the beans in the pan. Season with kosher salt and black pepper. Sauté for 5 minutes, or till the sauce has thickened, occasionally stirring, particularly at the end of the cooking process. Toast the bread and divide it between two plates just before the beans are cooked. Serve the beans on the side.

## Nutritional Facts

309 cals, Protein 13 g, Fats 7 g, Fiber 15 g, Carbs 41 g

## 2.16 Citrus Yogurt Parfait

Greek yoghurt is a high-protein snack that keeps you full for a long time. Opt for the plain version and add your tastes to avoid the added sugars found in some yogurts. Choose something sweet, something fruity, and something crunchy as a general rule. Honey, clementine and pistachios are used in this dish.

Preparation time: 5 minutes

Cooking time: 0 minutes

Serving: 4

**Ingredients**

- 3 cups plain nonfat Greek yogurt

- 1 teaspoon vanilla extract

- 28 clementine segments

- 4 teaspoons honey

- ¼ cup shelled unsalted dry-roasted chopped pistachios

**Instructions**

Combine yogurt and vanilla extract in a medium mixing basin. Pour a third of a cup of yogurt into each of the four parfait glasses. 1/2 teaspoon honey, 5 clementine segments, and 1/2 tablespoon pistachios on top. Add a quarter of the remaining yogurt, 1/2 teaspoon honey, 2 clementine segments, and 1/2 tablespoon pistachios to each parfait.

**Nutritional facts**

180cals, Protein 19 g, fats 4 g, Fiber 0 g, Carbs 40 g,

# 2.17 Cinnamon-Sugar Crisps

If there is no oil or butter in these chips, they are surprisingly crispy and tasty. Oversee them as they bake since they can quickly get burned around the edges.

Preparation time: 10 minutes

Cooking time: 15 minutes

Serving: 4

## Ingredients

- 1 tablespoon sugar

- 1 tablespoon water

- ¼ teaspoon ground cinnamon

- 2 8-inch flour tortillas

## Instructions

Preheat oven to 350°F.Put the sugar and cinnamon in a small bowl. Brush both sides of the tortillas with water and then sprinkle each side with the cinnamon-sugar mixture. Cut all tortillas into 12 wedges and arrange them on a cookie sheet in a single layer. Bake 15 minutes or until crisp. Let cookies cool \son a wire rack before serving.

## Nutritional facts

89cals, Protein 8 g, Fats 6 g, Fiber 20 g, Carbs 4.6 g,

## 2.18 Plantain Chips

Plantains may look like large bananas, but they have to be cooked before you eat them. They can also be a bit tough to peel, so use a sharp knife and be careful. They contain vitamins A and C, along with other nutrients.

Preparation time: 5 minutes

Cooking time: 3 minutes

Serving: 4

**Ingredients**

- 1 tablespoon olive oil
- 2 plantains (peeled and cut into ¼-inch dialogue slices)
- ¼ teaspoon salt
- ⅛ teaspoon ground red pepper

**Instructions**

Warm the oil in a skillet on the stove. Cook for 3 minutes on each side, or until plantain slices are golden and crispy. Take the pan out from the stove and sprinkle with salt and pepper before serving.

**Nutritional facts**

190cals, Protein 6 g, Fats 8.4 g, Fiber 4 g, Carbs 17 g,

## 2.19 Glazed Dried Fruit and Nuts

Think of this as trail mix kicked up a notch. It's fully customizable based on your preferences, so use any nuts, seeds, and dried fruit you want. Buy the nuts pre-chopped to save on prep time.

Preparation time: 5 minutes

Cooking time: 10 minutes

Serving: 4

**Ingredients**

- Cooking spray
- 1 teaspoon unsalted butter
- ¼ cup honey
- ¼ teaspoon salt
- ¼ cup slivered almonds
- ¼ cup chopped hazelnuts
- ¼ cup chopped pecans
- ¼ cup sunflower seeds
- ½ teaspoon ground cinnamon
- ¼ teaspoon ground cardamom
- 1 cup raisins
- Dash of ground cloves

## Instructions

Using parchment paper, line a baking pan. Set it aside after spraying it with cooking spray. Melt butter in a skillet on the stove. Cook for 2 minutes or till the honey l begins to bubble around the edges. Sunflower seeds, almonds, hazelnuts, pecans

**Nutritional facts**

190 cals, Protein 2 g, Fats 7 g, Fiber 10 g, Carbs 29 g

## 2.20 Sweet and Spicy Roasted Nuts

Roasted nuts are nothing new, but they stand out because of the addition of Indian spices like cardamom and cloves. Nuts are a fantastic snack since they're high in protein and heart-healthy unsaturated fat, so they'll keep you satisfied until your next meal. Like things a little spicier? Toss with a pinch of ground red pepper.

Preparation time: 9 minutes

Cooking time: 15 minutes

Serving: 4

**Ingredients**

- 1½ teaspoon packed brown sugar
- 1½ teaspoon honey
- 1 teaspoon canola oil
- ¾ teaspoon ground cinnamon
- ⅛ teaspoon salt
- ⅛ teaspoon ground cardamom
- ⅛ teaspoon ground cloves
- ¼ cup blanched almonds

- ¼ cup cashews

- ¼ cup hazelnuts

- Dash of ground pepper

## Instructions

Preheat oven to 350°F. Combine brown sugar, honey, oil, cinnamon, salt, cardamom, cloves, and pepper in a medium microwave-safe bowl. Stir after 30 seconds in the microwave. Add nuts to sugar mixture and toss to coat. Spread nuts equally on a baking sheet lined with parchment paper. Bake for 15 minutes or till it gets golden brown. Cool before serving.

## Nutritional facts

180cals, Protein 13 g, Fats, 8 g, Fiber 7 g, Carbs 22 g,

## 2.21 Peanut Butter Oatmeal Balls

These energizing nibbles are packed with fiber, protein, and healthy fat to keep you satisfied.

Preparation time: 10 minutes

Cooking time: 15 minutes

Serving: 4

## Ingredients

- ¼ cup old fashioned rolled oats

- 1 tablespoon chopped almonds

- 1 tablespoon ground flaxseed

- 1½ teaspoons chia seeds

- 1½ tablespoon creamy peanut butter

- 1 tablespoon honey

- 1 tablespoon mini chocolate chips

- ½ cup crushed peanuts for coating the balls

- Pinch of cinnamon

- Pinch of salt

- Dash of vanilla extract

## Instructions

Combine oats, chia seeds, almonds, flaxseeds, salt, and cinnamon in a large mixing dish. Microwave the peanut butter in a microwave-safe bowl for 20 to 30 seconds, or until melted; set aside to cool slightly. Mix in the honey and vanilla, then pour the peanut butter mixture over the oats. Once the mixture is combined and sticking together, fold in chocolate chips. Roll the dough into four balls with your hands, then roll them in crushed peanuts.

## Nutritional facts

260cals, Protein 4 g, Fats 8 g, Fiber 2 g, Carbs 10 g,

# Chapter 3 Shakes and Soups Recipes

Shakes may be a great way to stay on track by serving as a meal substitute. Soups, on the other hand, are both appetizing and satisfying. You may take one part to work for lunch and keep the other portions in the fridge or freezer for a few days. Soups may be your fast-day buddy.

## 3.1 Shakes

### 3.1.1 Ice Berry Shake

For this refreshing smoothie, use whatever frozen fruit you choose. Make sure your food processor is capable of crushing ice.

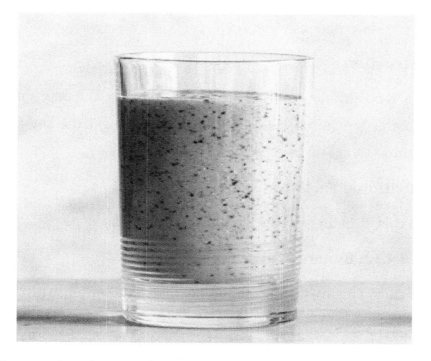

Preparation time: 5 minutes

Cook time: 0 minutes

Serving: 1

**Ingredients**

- Greek yogurt (25g)

- Semi-skimmed milk, 75 mL

- 40g frozen mixed berries strawberries, blueberries, etc.

- 1/2 medium peeled and coarsely chopped bananas (about 50g)

- 1 tablespoon porridge oats

- 5 g almond flour

- 2 tablespoons water (cool)

**Instructions**

In a food grinder, add all of the ingredients and mix until smooth. If required, add additional water to get the smooth texture.

**Nutritional Facts**

190 cals, Protein 5 g, Fats 4 g, Fiber 2.3 g, Carbs 22 g,

### 3.1.2 Banana Nutty Shake

For this creamy-tasting smoothie, use nut butter with no added sugar.

Preparation time: 5 minutes

Cook time: 0 minutes

Serving: 1

## Ingredients

- 20g live Greek yoghurt (full fat)

- semi-skimmed milk (100 mL)

- 1/2 medium bananas, peeled and coarsely chopped (about 50g peeled weight)

- 15g nut butter without sugar made from cashews or almonds

- 2 tablespoons water (cool)

## Instruction

In a food grinder, add all of the ingredients and mix until smooth. If required, add additional water to get the smooth texture.

## Nutritional Facts

214 cals, Protein 17 g, Fats 1 g, Fiber 2 g, Carbs 8 g

### 3.1.3 Strawberry and Chocolate Shake

A chocolatey hit that is both tasty and filling.

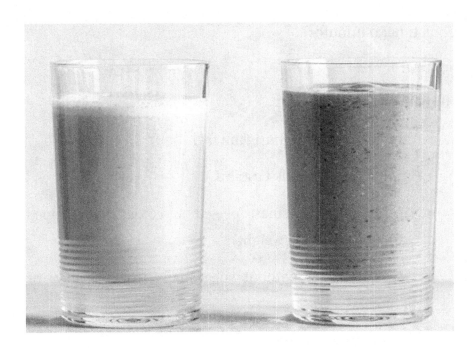

Preparation time: 10 minutes

Cook time: 0 minutes

Serving: 1

**Ingredients**

- semi-skimmed milk (100 mL)

- 25 g live Greek yogurt (full fat)

- 100g strawberries (fresh or frozen)

- giant porridge oats (15g)

- 1 date with a soft pit

- a teaspoon of cocoa powder

- 2 tbsp water (cool)

## Instructions

In a food grinder, add all of the ingredients and mix until smooth. If required, add additional water to get the smooth texture.

## Nutritional Facts

195 cals, Protein 12 g, Fats, 0.8 g, Fiber 3.7 g, Carbs 13 g.

### 3.1.4 Minted Cucumber and Avocado Shake

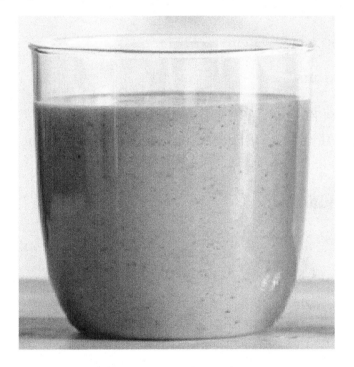

A smooth, velvety shake with a touch of mint.

Preparation time: 15 minutes

Cook time: 0 minutes

Serving: 1

## Ingredients

- 1/2 medium avocados, chopped, skinned, and cut into quarters (about 75 grams)

- 200 g thickly sliced cucumber

- 25 g leaves of young spinach

- 15g full-fat live Greek yogurt

- Fresh mint leaves (12grams)

- 100 ml ice water

## Instructions

In a food grinder, add all of the ingredients and mix until smooth. If required, add additional water to get the smooth texture.

## Nutritional Facts

205 cals, Protein 3 g, Fats 8 g, Fiber 5 g, Carbs 14 g

### 3.1.5 Cashew, Carrot and Orange Shake

A smooth, velvety shake with a touch of mint.

This results in a citrusy drink with a bright orange color. Make sure your food mixer is capable of handling the carrot slices.

Preparation time: 20 minutes

Cook time: 0 minutes

Serving: 1

## Ingredients

- 1/2 medium-size orange, skinned and cut into rough pieces

- 1/2 medium carrots (about 170g), trimmed and thinly sliced

- 15 g cashew nut butter or hazelnut butter with no added sugar

- 125 milliliters of cold water

## Instructions

In a food grinder, add all of the ingredients and mix until smooth. If required, add additional water to get the smooth texture.

## Nutritional Facts

215 cals, Protein 3 g, Fats 1 g, Fiber 4.8 g, Carbs 42 g

### 3.1.6 Ginger Shake

This lovely green shake is made with a crisp green apple that provides fiber and flavor. If you like, use a red-skinned apple.

Preparation time: 20 minutes

Cook time: 0 minutes

Serving: 1

Ingredients

- 1 quartered green apple

- 1/2 medium courgette, chopped and finely chopped (about 65g)

- 8g peeled and finely chopped fresh root ginger

- 1/2 tsp turmeric powder

- 10 grams of mixed seeds (sunflower, pumpkin and flax)

- 2 teaspoons extra-virgin olive oil

- 100 mL ice water

## Instructions

In a food grinder, add all of the ingredients and mix until smooth. If required, add additional water to get the smooth texture.

## Nutritional Facts

196 cals, Protein 4.2 g, Fats 3 g, Fiber 13 g, Carbs 15g

### 3.1.7 Gazpacho Shake

It is delicious served chilled with a few ice cubes.

Preparation time: 15 minutes

Cook time: 0 minutes

Serving: 1

## Ingredients

- cucumber, 100g, coarsely chopped

- 2 to 3 healthy vine tomatoes, cut into quarters (about 125g)

- 1/2 red pepper, without seed and chopped

- 1/2 red pepper, without seed and chopped

- 25 g Greek yogurt (full fat)

- 10 g almond flour

- 1 tablespoon pureed tomatoes

- 1 teaspoon extra-virgin olive oil

- 2 tablespoons water (cool)

- to taste with salt and black pepper

**Instructions**

In a food grinder, add all of the ingredients and mix until smooth. If required, add additional water to get the smooth texture.

**Nutritional Facts**

192 cals, Protein 3 g, Fats 0.8 g, Fiber 3 g, Carbs 19 g.

### 3.1.8 Chai Smoothie

Black tea, cinnamon, black pepper, and other herbs spices are combined in chai tea. It originated in India but is now so popular it can be found in most grocery stores.

Preparation time: 40 minutes

Cooking time: 0 minutes

Serving: 1

**Ingredients**

- ½ cup boiling water

- 4 chai tea bags

- ¼ cup sugar

- 2 cups ice

- ½ cup 1% milk

**Instructions**

Combine boiling water, sugar, and chai tea bags in a small bowl. Cover and set aside for 5 minutes to steep. Discard tea bags, then refrigerate tea for 30 minutes or until thoroughly chilled. Place tea, ice, and milk in a blender and process until smooth. Serve immediately.

**Nutritional facts**

246cals, Protein 6 g, Fats 0 g, Fiber 0 g, Carbs 20 g

## 3.2 Soups

### 3.2.1 Bean Soup with Pesto and Kale

It is super-quick and simple to make, and it tastes fantastic with the fresh herbs pesto on top. You may use whichever beans you choose as long as the quantity remains the same.

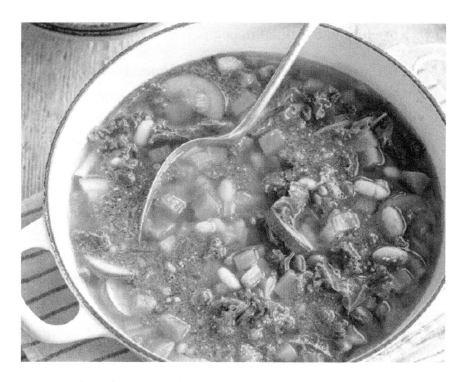

Preparation time: 15 minutes

Cook time: 20 minutes

Serving: 4

**Ingredients**

- 2 tablespoons extra virgin olive oil

- 1 medium peeled and chopped fresh onion

- 1 celery stick, roughly cut into 1 cm pieces

- 2 medium carrots, peeled and chopped into 1 cm slices

- 1 medium courgette, half lengthwise and sliced into 1cm thick slices

- 400g drained cannellini beans

- Borlotti beans in a can (400g) or drained beans

- 1 cube of vegetable or chicken broth

- 75g thickly sliced kale or dark green cabbage, with rough stems removed

- 60 g pesto (fresh basil)

## Instructions

In a large size nonstick saucepan, heat the oil and gently cook the onion, celery, carrots, and courgette for 10 minutes, stirring periodically. Add the beans, stock cube, and 1.2 liters of water to the pan and stir to dissolve. Put the kale or cabbage to a low simmer. Cook, occasionally stirring, for 5–7 minutes, or until the veggies are soft. Season with sea salt and freshly ground black pepper, then spoon into hot bowls and top with pesto.

## Nutritional Facts

249cals, Protein 7 g, Fats 14.5 g, Fiber 8 g, Carbs 18.5 g

### 3.2.2 Broccoli Cheese Soup

A hearty, warming soup that's also beneficial for your gut microbes.

Preparation time: 20 minutes

Cook time: 20 minutes

Serving: 4

## Ingredients

- 1 tablespoon olive or canola oil

- 1 peeled and coarsely chopped medium onion

- 1 broccoli head (about 400g) coarsely cut, including the stem

- 1 cube of vegetable or chicken stock

- 75g blue cheese (Roquefort, for example)

## Instructions

Take a large nonstick saucepan, heat the oil, add the onion, and cook for 5 minutes, or till it becomes softened, stirring often. Put the broccoli and top with a crumbled stock cube. Bring 1 liter of water to a boil in a separate pot. Slow down the heat to low and cook, turning regularly, for 10 minutes, or till the broccoli is very soft. Take off the heat and mix until smooth with a hand mixer or in a spice grinder after cooling somewhat. Bring to the heat, add the majority of the cheese, and season to taste. Warm through gently, if necessary, with a splash of water, before dishing with the remaining cheese scattered on top.

## Nutritional Facts

158 cals, Protein 8.5 g, Fats 10 g, Fiber 5 g, Carbs 6 g

### 3.3.3 Bean and Spinach Soup

This soup, made using items you may find in your pantry and freezer, will keep you going all day. Harissa is a spicy red pepper and chili paste found in the supermarket's World Foods area.

Preparation time: 20 minutes

Cook time: 25 minutes

Serving: 4

**Ingredients**

- 1 tablespoon extra-virgin olive oil
- 1 medium onion, peeled and cut finely
- 1 big peeled and smashed garlic clove
- 1 tsp cumin powder
- 1 tablespoon of harissa paste
- 400g chopped tomatoes in a can
- one cannellini bean (400g) drained and washed
- 1 cube of vegetable stock
- 200g spinach, frozen

**Instructions**

Take a large nonstick saucepan, heat the oil, add the onion, and cook for 5 minutes, stirring until it becomes softened. Cook for a few moments more, constantly stirring, after adding the

garlic, cumin, and harissa paste. Crumble the stock cube over the tomatoes and cannellini beans in the pan. Stir in 500ml water and the frozen spinach. Bring the liquid to a low simmer (it may take a while since the spinach has to defrost), then cook for 10 minutes, stirring occasionally and adding a little more water if necessary. To serve, season with salt and freshly ground black pepper.

Nutritional Facts

200cals, Protein 10.5 g, Fats 5 g, Fiber 9 g, Carbs 22.5 g

### 3.3.4 Instant Noodle Soup

A tasty Asian-inspired soup that's perfect for a lunch on the run.

Preparation time: 20 minutes

Cook time: 30 minutes

Serving: 2

**Ingredients**

- 50g soba buckwheat noodles or 50g dry whole wheat noodles

- 4 tablespoons miso paste

- 20g peeled and coarsely grated fresh root ginger

- 2 tablespoons soy sauce (dark)

- Depending on size, 4–6 chestnut mushrooms

- one big handful of very finely cut young spinach leaves (about 75g)

- 4 trimmed and thinly sliced spring onions

- 1/2 teaspoons dried chili flakes, crushed

- 25g coarsely chopped roasted cashew nuts

- 2 heaping handfuls of coarsely chopped fresh coriander leaves

**Instructions**

Bring a pot half-full of water to a boil. Return to a boil, add the noodles and simmer for 3–4 minutes, or according to the package directions, until tender. Using a strainer, strain the noodles and rinse them under cold running water. Drain thoroughly. In two big heatproof jars, divide the miso paste, ginger, and soy sauce. On top of the mushrooms, layer the cooked noodles, spinach, spring onions, chili flakes, cashews, and coriander in the following order: cooked noodles, spinach, spring onions, chili flakes, cashews, and coriander. Cover and refrigerate. When ready to serve, fill each jar halfway with 250–300ml freshly boiled water (about a cup full). About midway through the ingredients, the water should increase. Allow 2 minutes for the veggies to soften and the noodles to cook before covering loosely. Stir thoroughly, then set aside for another 1–2 minutes before serving.

## Nutritional Facts

210cals, Protein 9 g, Fats 7 g, Fiber 2.5 g, Carbs 26.5 g

### 3.3.5 Creamy Mushroom Soup

A decadent, creamy mushroom soup that's surprisingly simple to prepare and low in calories. Don't miss any of the cooking phases; they all contribute to the final flavor.

Preparation time: 20 minutes

Cook time: 30 minutes

Serving: 2

## Ingredients

- 1 tablespoon olive oil

- 1 peeled and coarsely chopped big onion

- 300 g sliced chestnut mushrooms or any other mushrooms

- 2 big peeled and smashed garlic cloves

- 1 cube of vegetable or chicken broth

- 75 milliliters of full-fat milk

## Instructions

Take a large nonstick saucepan, heat the oil, add the onion and cook, often turning, for 5 minutes, or it becomes softened and lightly browned. Sauté for 5 minutes, occasionally stirring, after adding the mushrooms and garlic. Allowing the garlic to roast will result in a bitter flavor. Pour 600ml water over the stock cube and crumble it. Season with a generous amount of ground black pepper and a pinch of sea salt. Return to a fire, lower to low heat and cook, stirring periodically, for 10 minutes. Turn off the heat and mix until smooth with a hand mixer or in a spice grinder after cooling somewhat. Transfer the pan to the fire and season to taste with the milk. To obtain your desired consistency, add a bit more milk or water and reheat well before serving.

## Nutritional Facts

68cals, Protein 3 g, Fats 4 g, Fiber 1.5 g, Carbs 4 g

### 3.3.6 Chicken and Pea Soup

This easy soup is a fantastic way to use up leftover roast chicken or turkey. Use a good-quality chicken broth cube instead of fresh stock if you don't have any on hand. If desired, add finely chopped parsley or tarragon leaves.

Preparation time: 20 minutes

Cook time: 30 minutes

Serving: 4

Ingredients

- 1 tablespoon olive oil

- 1 peeled and coarsely chopped small onion

- 150g cooked leftover chicken, coarsely chopped

- 500 milliliters of fresh chicken stock

- 150g peas, frozen

## Instructions

Take a nonstick saucepan, heat the oil, and then add the onion and cook, often turning, for 3–4 minutes, or until softened. Sprinkle with ground black pepper and bring to a boil with the chicken, stock, and peas. Cook, stirring periodically, for 5 minutes. Serve immediately in two hot bowls.

## Nutritional Facts

280cals, Protein 29.5 g, Fats 12.5 g, Fiber 4.5 g, Carbs 10 g

### 3.3.7 Chicken and Lentil Soup

The lentils and spinach in this soup provide a lot of fiber, making it quite satisfying.

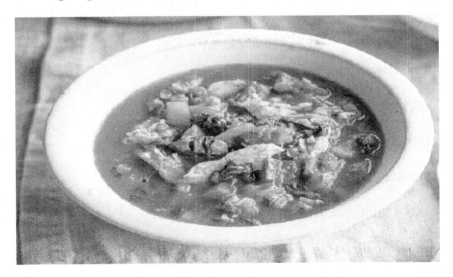

Preparation time: 20 minutes

Cook time: 30 minutes

Serving: 4

## Ingredients

- 1 tablespoon coconut or olive oil

- 1 medium peeled and coarsely chopped onion

- 1 pepper, deseeded and sliced into 1.5cm cubes, any color

- 2 tablespoon curry powder (medium)

- 400 g chopped tomatoes in a can

- 1 cube of chicken stock

- 50g red split lentils, dry

- 225g spinach, frozen

- 200g cooked chicken, cut roughly

- Serve with lemon wedges.

## Instructions

Take a large nonstick saucepan, heat the oil, add the onion and pepper, and cook for 5 minutes, or until it becomes softened. Cook for a few more seconds after adding the curry powder. Bring to a boil with the tomatoes. Stir for a few minutes more, then crumble in the chicken broth cube and 1 liter of water.

Wash the lentils with fresh water and place them in the pan with the frozen spinach. Bring to low heat. Season with a generous amount of crushed black pepper and a pinch of sea salt. Cook, occasionally stirring, for 10 minutes. Cook and occasionally stir for at least 8 to 10 minutes, or until the lentils are mushy and the spinach has thawed. If the soup becomes too sticky, add a little bit more water. Season to taste, then serve in deep dishes with lemon wedges for squeezing over the top.

**Nutritional Facts**

223 cals, Protein 20.5 g, Fats 8 g, Fiber 4.5 g, Carbs 15.5 g

### 3.3.8 Tomato Soup

A quick lunch or dinner with the addition of beans to make it more filling.

Preparation time: 10 minutes

Cook time: 20 minutes

Serving: 2

**Ingredients**

- 400g chopped tomatoes in a can
- Cannellini beans, half a 400g can drain
- 2 clipped and coarsely chopped spring onions
- 30g Greek yogurt (full fat).

- 6 big basil leaves, with more to serve (if desired)

- 1 tablespoon olive oil

- 1 tablespoon tomato puree

## Instructions

In a blender, combine all ingredients, sprinkle with sea salt and plenty of ground black pepper, and mix until smooth. Transfer to a nonstick saucepan, add enough water to get your desired consistency and gently cook through. Salt to taste and serve in bowls or cups, garnished with basil leaves if desired.

## Nutritional Facts

192cals, Protein 8 g, Fats 7.5 g, Fiber 6.5 g, Carbs 20 g

# Chapter 4: Lunch

## 4.1 Roast Chicken Thighs with Lemon

This succulent, herb-infused chicken goes well with a large green and colored leaf salad prepared with salad dressing or a large portion of freshly cooked veggies. It's also fantastic at the BBQ.

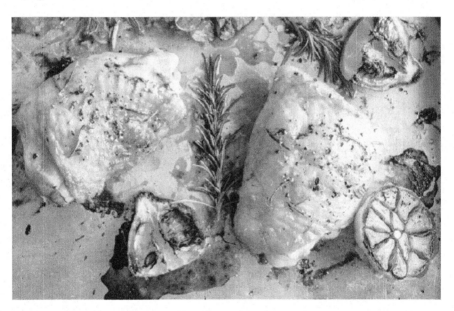

Preparation time: 5 hours

Cooking time: 1 hour

Serving: 2

**Ingredients**

- 4 chicken thighs (bone-in) (each around 150g)

- 1 to 2 lemons, 1 quartered, 1 with juice (about 2 tbsp.) (optional)

- 1 tablespoon extra-virgin olive oil

- 2 tablespoons fresh thyme leaves or 2–3 rosemary sprigs, roughly chopped (or 1 teaspoon dried herbs)

- 1 garlic bulb, halved (optional)

## Instructions

Preheat your oven to 200°C if you're going to cook the chicken right away. Combine the chicken, lemon juice, and oil in a mixing basin. Season it with sea salt and plenty of ground black pepper after adding the thyme or rosemary. Toss everything together thoroughly. Cover and marinate in the fridge for a minimum of 1 hour and up to 4 hours if you have time.

Bake the chicken for 15 minutes, skin-side up, in a roasting tin with the herbs and quartered lemon, if using. Take the tin out of the oven and cook at least 20 to 25 minutes, or until the chicken is gently browned, tender, and cooked through.

### Nutritional facts

385 cals, Protein 58 g, Fats 17 g, Fiber 0 g, Carbs 0 g

## 4.2 Chicken Goujons with Parmesan Crumb

Preparation time: 1 hours

Cooking time: 45 minutes

Serving: 2

Tender chicken breasts coated in a crunchy golden Parmesan crust. Warm with a large mixed salad and Simple salad dressing, steamed sliced courgette, or a generous serving of mange tout.

## Ingredients

- 1 medium egg

- 50 gram Parmesan, finely grated

- 25g quick-cook polenta

- ½ teaspoon. dried thyme

- ½ teaspoon paprika

- 2 boneless chicken breast fillets (around 400g), each cut into 4 to 5 thin strips

- lemon wedges, to serve

## Instructions

Preheat the oven to 200 degrees. Use the nonstick baking paper to line a big baking tray. Take a medium mixing bowl, whisk the egg until it is completely silky. Take a separate bowl, mix all the ingredients, including Parmesan, polenta, thyme, and paprika, with some salt and a crushed grind of black pepper. Spread out half of the mixture on a large plate. Dip the chicken strips in the egg, one at a time, and then in the Parmesan crumb. When the initial batch of crumbs is gone, add more to the plate. Place the

goujons on the baking sheet and bake for 12–14 minutes, or until crisp and golden brown. Serve with a squeeze of lemon, divided between two dishes.

**Nutritional facts**

399 cals, Protein 62 g, Fats 13 g, Fiber 0.5 g, Carbs 9 g

## 4.3 One-pot roast chicken

A one-pot chicken recipe that's great for a family supper.

Preparation time: 1 hour

Cooking time: 1 hours 30 minutes

Serving: 4

**Ingredients**

- 2 smoked bacon rashers, cut into 2cm strips

- 1 medium peeled and sliced onion

- 1 chicken, medium (around 1.6kg)

- 1 tablespoon. extra virgin olive oil

- 150g trimmed young carrots

- 150g peeled and trimmed baby parsnips

- 200 mL chicken stock

- 100ml dry white wine or more broth

- 1 tablespoon thyme leaves, fresh

- 12 teaspoon dried thyme (optional)

- 200g peas, frozen

## Instructions

Preheat the oven to 200 degrees. In a medium flame-proof casserole, combine the bacon and onion, then top with the chicken. Season with sea salt and powdered black pepper after drizzling with oil. Roast the chicken for 30 minutes, uncovered, until golden brown.

Take the casserole from the oven, transfer the chicken to a platter, and stir in the carrots and parsnips. Pour in the stock and wine, if desired, and top with thyme, if desired. Cover the casserole with a lid and bake for a further 45–55 minutes, or till the veggies get soft and the chicken is cooked correctly. Carefully transfer the chicken to a hot plate. Place the dish on the stovetop and skim off any fat that has surfaced. Bring the liquid to a boil after adding the peas (take care as the pan will be very hot). 2–3 minutes, or until the pan juices have been reduced by half. Season with salt and pepper to taste. Carve the chicken into small pieces and serve with the veggies and cooking liquor in deep dishes or bowls.

**Nutritional facts**

460 cals, Protein 44.5 g, Fats 18.5 g, Fiber 8.5 g, Carbs 20g

## 4.4 Simple chicken casserole

Delicious comfort meal for a family dinner that can be reheated the next day or frozen for further use. Serve with vegetables, such as cabbage, broccoli, green beans, or kale that have just been cooked.

Preparation time: 40 minutes

Cooking time: 1 hour

Serving: 4

**Ingredients**

- 2 tbsp. olive oil

- 6 boneless, skinless chicken thighs (around 600g), quartered

- 2 smoked back bacon rashers, cut into roughly 2cm strips

- 1 large onion, peeled and finely sliced

- 150g button mushrooms, halved or sliced if large

- 1 × 400g can chopped tomatoes

- 3 medium carrots, trimmed and cut into roughly 1cm slices

- 1 chicken stock cube

- 1 tsp. mixed dried herbs

## Instructions

Preheat the oven to 200 degrees. In a flame-proof casserole dish, heat the oil over medium heat. Season the chicken, bacon, onion, and mushrooms with a pinch of sea salt and plenty of ground black pepper, then cook, frequently stirring, for 6–8 minutes, until the chicken is browned on all sides' onion is gently browned.

Combine the tomatoes, carrots, crumbled stock cube, and dry herbs in a large mixing bowl. Pour in 400ml cold water and mix thoroughly. Bring to a low simmer, cover and bake for 40 minutes, or until the chicken is cooked through.

### Nutritional facts

303 cals, Protein 36 g, Fats 12.5 g, Fiber 4 g, Carbs 9 g

# 4.5 Chicken Wrapped in Parma Ham

In our house, this is a trendy dish. Serve with a large mixed salad as a side dish.

Preparation time: 30 minutes

Cooking time: 45 minutes

Serving: 4

### Ingredients

- 4 boneless, chicken breasts each around 150g

- 4 slices Parma ham or prosciutto

- 2 tablespoon olive oil

- 1 medium onion, peeled and finely chopped

- 2 garlic cloves, peeled and crushed

- Can chopped tomatoes 400 grams or 500g passata

- 1 teaspoon dried oregano

- 200 grams young spinach leaves

- 25 grams Parmesan, finely grated

## Instructions

Cover the chicken with a sheet of cling film and place it aboard. Flatten with a rolling pin until it's about 2cm thick. Pack each breast chicken in a slice of Parma ham and season with sea salt and powdered black pepper.

In a large nonstick frying pan or shallow flame-proof casserole dish, heat 1 tablespoon of the oil. Fry the wrapped chicken for 3–4 minutes on each side over medium heat or lightly browned. Place on a plate to cool.

Cook the leftover oil in the pan with the onion for 5 minutes, then add the garlic and cook for several more minutes.

Add the chopped tomatoes or passata, oregano, 300ml water, and spinach (the pan will look full). Bring to a gentle simmer, stirring regularly, for 2–3 minutes, or until the spinach is very tender. Season the sauce with salt and pepper.

Put the chicken in the saucepan again and nestle it into the sauce. Simmer for 18–20 minutes, or until the chicken is soft and thoroughly cooked, stirring occasionally. If necessary, add a splash of water. To serve, top with a sprinkling of Parmesan cheese.

**Nutritional facts**

321 cals, Protein 44.5 g, Fats 11 g, Fiber 3.5 g, Carbs 10 g

## 4.6 Easy Chicken Tagine

A filling Moroccan-inspired casserole with lovely fiber-rich chickpeas. Don't be frightened off by the enormous list of ingredients; after the chicken has been cooked, it's a simple toss-it-in-the-oven recipe. Serve with a big salad or a large number of green beans.

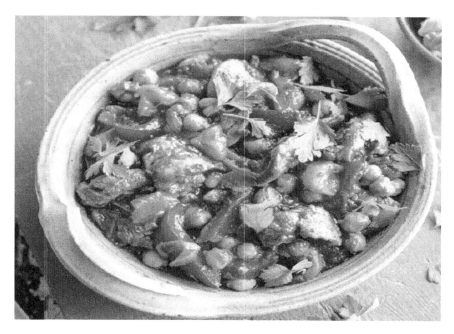

Preparation time: 45 minutes

Cooking time: 1 hour

Serving: 2

## Ingredients

- 2 tbsp. olive oil
- 1 medium onion, peeled and thinly sliced
- 1½ tsp. ground cumin
- ¼ tsp. ground cinnamon
- 3 boneless, skinless chicken thighs (around 300g)
- 1½ teaspoon ground coriander
- 1 red pepper deseeded cut into 3cm chunks)
- 1 can chopped tomatoes (400 g )
- 1 chicken stock cube
- 1 can washed chickpea (around 130g drained weight)
- 4 dried apricots (around 25g), roughly chopped
- Fresh coriander or parsley leaves chopped, to serve

## Instructions

Preheat your oven to 200 degrees. In a medium flame-proof casserole, heat the oil over medium heat. Add the onion and chicken and cook, frequently turning, for 6–8 minutes, or until the onion is lightly browned. Season with the spices and heat for a few more seconds, stirring constantly. Combine the pepper, tomatoes, chickpeas, apricots, and crumbled stock cube in a large mixing bowl. Bring to a simmer with 250ml water, a pinch of sea salt, and lots of ground black pepper. Cook for 45 minutes in the oven, covered until the chicken is cooked and the sauce has thickened. To serve, garnish with coriander or parsley.

**Nutritional facts**

447 cals, Protein 41 g, Fats 17 g, Fiber 10 g, Carbs 27g

## 4.7 Chinese-Style Drumsticks

Drumsticks are baked in the oven, but they're also fantastic on the grill. Serve with a large mixed salad or steamed pak choi or spring greens.

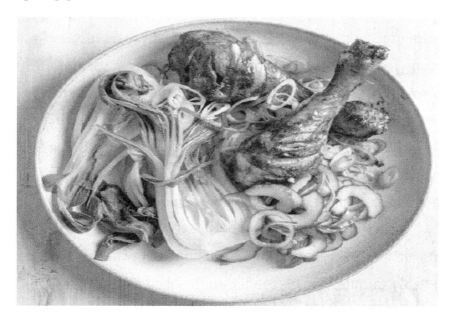

Preparation time: 40 minutes

Cooking time: 45 minutes

Serving: 4

## Ingredients

- 2 teaspoon Chinese spice powder

- 4 tablespoon soya sauce

- Sesame oil 2 teaspoon

- 2 garlic cloves skinned and crushed

- 8 chicken thighs

- 2 spring onions finely sliced (optional)

## Instructions

Take a large mixing bowl, combine the five-spice soy sauce, sesame oil, and garlic. Add 2–3 slashes through the thickest section of each chicken drumstick to the marinade. Mix thoroughly. Cover and marinate for a minimum of 20 to 30 minutes, preferably several hours, in the fridge, turning regularly. Preheat your oven to 220 degrees Celsius. Using foil, line a large baking tray. Bake the drumsticks for 20 minutes on the preheated sheet, reserving any remaining marinade in the bowl. Take the chicken out from the oven and baste it with the leftover marinade before putting it into the oven for another 10 to 20 minutes, or till tender and cooked through. If using, garnish with spring onions before serving.

**Nutritional facts**

238 cals, Protein 33 g, Fats 10.5 g, Fiber 0 g, Carbs 3g

## 4.8 Chicken Tikka Masala

A healthier version of a favorite curry that tastes just as good
as takeout. Make sure you use a high-quality tikka curry paste.
Serve with cauliflower rice or steamed greens.

Preparation time: 4 hours

Cooking time: 1 hour

Serving: 4

### Ingredients

- 1 tablespoon tikka curry paste

- 4 tablespoon full-fat live Greek yogurt

- 2 boneless chicken breasts around 350g cut into
  roughly 3cm chunks

- 1 tablespoon coconut oil

- fresh coriander, to serve (optional)

- ½ red chili, sliced for serving

### For masala sauce

- 1 tablespoon coconut oil

- 1 medium onion peeled and finely chopped

- 2 garlic cloves, peeled and crushed

- 15-gram fresh ginger, peeled and finely grated

- 2 tablespoon tikka curry paste

- 1 tablespoon tomato purée

## Instructions

Combine the curry paste, yogurt, and 2 liberal pinches of sea salt in a mixing dish. Mix in the chicken until it is evenly coated. Cover and marinate for at least 1 hour, preferably longer or overnight, in the fridge.

Make the sauce fifteen minutes before you're ready to serve. In a nonstick saucepan, heat the oil on medium heat. Then add the onion and sauté for 5 minutes, or until softened, then add the garlic, ginger, and curry paste and continue to cook for another 112 minutes. Fill the pan halfway with water, then add the tomato purée and heat to a simmer. Cook for a minimum of 5 to 7 minutes, and then remove the pan from the heat and blitz the sauce with a hand blender. Remove from the equation. In a frying pan, heat the oil (remaining) over medium-high heat and cook the marinated chicken for at least 3 minutes, or until lightly browned, flipping frequently. Bring the prepared sauce to a simmer in the pan. Cook and stir regularly, for 3–4 minutes, or until the chicken is thoroughly cooked. If the sauce becomes too thick, add a drop of water. To serve with chopped coriander and chili if used.

## Nutritional facts

427 cals, Protein 46 g, Fats 21 g, Fiber 4 g, Carbs 11.5 g

## 4.9 Chicken, Pepper and Chorizo Bake

A simple chicken bake full of healthy Mediterranean ingredients and wonderful Spanish flavors. Serve with a large leafy salad.

Preparation time: 1 hour

Cooking time: 1 hour

Serving: 2

**Ingredients**

- 1 red onion chopped and cut into 12 wedges

- 4 medium tomatoes, quartered

- 2 peppers (any color), deseeded and cut into roughly 3cm chunks

- 1 tablespoon olive oil

- 4 boneless, skinless chicken thighs (around 400g)

- ½ teaspoon smoked paprika

- 25g chorizo, diced

**Instructions**

Heat the oven to 200 degrees. In a large baking dish, combine the onions, tomatoes, and peppers. Drizzle the oil over the top and mix lightly. Put the chicken thighs in the middle of the vegetables.

Roast for 30 minutes after sprinkling with paprika, seasoning with sea salt and plenty of ground black pepper. Tale the tray out from the oven, add the chorizo, and cook for an additional 5 to 10 minutes, or till the chorizo is hot and browning.

**Nutritional facts**

421 cals, Protein 47 g, Fats 17 g, Fiber 7 g, Carbs 17 g

## 4.10 Easy Jerk Chicken

Juicy, spicy Caribbean chicken that's great on the grill or in the oven. Serve with a large mixed salad as a side dish.

Preparation time: 50 minutes

Cooking time: 1 hour

Serving: 4

**Ingredients**

- 8 boneless, skinless chicken thighs (around 800g)
- For the marinade
- 1 medium onion, peeled and roughly chopped
- 2 garlic cloves, peeled
- 1 scotch bonnet chili or 1 tsp. crushed dried chili flakes
- juice 1 large lime, plus extra wedges to serve

- 2 tbsp. dark soy sauce

- 1 tsp. dried thyme

- 1 tsp. ground allspice

## Instructions

To prepare a paste, blitz all of the marinade ingredients in a food processor with a pinch of sea salt and plenty of ground black pepper. Alternatively, grate the onion, crush the garlic, and finely chop the chili before mixing the remaining ingredients. (After touching the chili, wash your hands well.) In a large mixing basin, combine the marinade ingredients. With a knife, carefully score the thickest part of the bird. Add the chicken to the marinade, swirl well, then cover and marinate for at least 2 hours or overnight in the refrigerator. Preheat the oven to 200 degrees Celsius. Using foil, line a baking tray. Brush the chicken with the marinade and place it on the prepared tray. Cook for 25 minutes, or until the chicken is lightly browned and entirely done. Lime wedges are provided for squeezing over the top.

## Nutritional facts

241 cals, Protein 42 g, Fats 6 g, Fiber 1 g, Carbs 4.5 g

# 4.11 Satay Chicken

Even on a fast day, you may have this delectable and hearty satay sauce as a dip or drizzled now that nuts are back on the menu. We like to cook these on a ridged grill, and you can also cook on the grill or the barbecue. It's beautiful cold and makes for a great take-along lunch. Serve with a mixed salad on the side.

Preparation time: 40 minutes

Cooking time: 1 hour

Serving: 4

## Ingredients

- 1 tbsp. coconut or rapeseed oil

- Juice 1 lime (around 2 tbsp.)

- ½ tsp. crushed dried chili flakes

- 2 tsp. dark soy sauce

- lime wedges, to serve

- 3 boneless, skinless chicken breasts (175g), cut into 16 long, thin strips

- 1 green chili (optional)

## For the satay sauce

- 60g no-added-sugar crunchy peanut butter (around 4 tbsp)

- 1 tbsp. dark soy sauce

- 15g root ginger (peeled and finely grated)

## Instructions

If using coconut oil, slowly melt it in a small saucepan before pouring it into a medium mixing bowl. Add the lime juice, chili flakes, soy sauce, and black pepper to taste. Mix thoroughly. Toss in the chicken strips and thoroughly combine everything. Using the skewers, thread the chicken strips on. Working fast is necessary since the lime juice will begin to 'cook' the chicken. The coconut oil will start to harden.

Cook the chicken for at least 3 to 5 minutes more on each side, depending on thickness, on a large, lightly greased griddle or nonstick frying pan over medium-high heat or until lightly browned and cooked through. Meanwhile, make the satay sauce by combining the peanut butter, 4 tablespoons water, soy sauce, and shredded ginger in a small saucepan.

Heat on low heat, stirring regularly until the peanut butter softens and the mixture thickens and becomes glossy. If necessary, add a bit more soy sauce or water to taste. In individual dipping bowls or drizzled over the chicken, serve with lime wedges, chili, if using, and the warm sauce.

## Nutritional facts

264 cals, Protein 36 g, Fats 12 g, Fiber 1 g, Carbs 3g

## 4.12 Turkey fajitas

Turkey is a substitute for chicken, and iceberg lettuce is ideal for this delectable Mexican-style filling.

Preparation time: 50 minutes

Cooking time: 1 hour 30 minutes

Serving: 4

### Ingredients

- 1 iceberg lettuce

- 1 tablespoon olive oil

- 400g thin turkey breast steaks finely sliced into thin strips

- 1 medium onion roughly chopped and cut into 12 small pieces

- 2 peppers, 1 red and 1 yellow, and roughly thinly sliced

- 1 teaspoon hot smoked paprika

- 1 teaspoon ground cumin

- 1 teaspoon coriander

- Fresh coriander leaves roughly chopped to serve

- 100g full-fat live Greek yogurt

- lime wedges, to serve

## Instructions

Put the lettuce over and cut around the stalk end with a little knife to separate the leaves. At least eight leaves should be carefully peeled, removed, washed, and drained. Arrange the leaves on a serving dish or board. Cook the turkey, onion, and peppers in a large nonstick frying pan over medium heat for at least 5 to 10 minutes, or till the turkey is cooked and the veggies are softened and gently browned tossing frequently. Stir in the spices and simmer for another 1–2 minutes. Season with a pinch of salt and a generous amount of freshly ground black pepper. Transfer the pan to the table or a hot dish and top with a generous amount of coriander. Fill the leaves with heated turkey, yogurt, and lime wedges for squeezing.

## Nutritional facts

195 cals, Protein 28 g, Fats 5 g, Fiber 3 g, Carbs 7.5 g

# 4.13 Perfect Pulled Pork

This juicy, zingy pork reheats well and may be eaten the next day as well. Serve in lettuce wraps with diced cornichons and Little Gem or romaine lettuce leaves.

Preparation time: 5 hours

Cooking time: 1 hour 30 minutes

Serving: 6

## Ingredients

- 1kg pork shoulder joint, rind on
- For the marinade
- 45g tomato purée (around 3 tbsp)
- 30g chipotle paste (around 2 tbsp)
- juice 2 large oranges
- juice 2 limes
- 1 tsp. flaked sea salt
- 1 tsp. ground cumin
- 1 tsp. ground allspice
- 1 tsp. coarsely ground black pepper

## Instructions

In a large non-metallic mixing basin, whisk the tomato purée, chipotle paste, orange and lime juice, salt, and spices to form the marinade. Please remove any remaining string from the pork and place it in the marinade. Turn the pork several times until it is well coated, then cover and marinate overnight in the refrigerator.

Preheat the oven to 170 degrees Celsius. In a medium casserole, combine the pork and marinade, cover, and bake for 3 hours, or until the pork breaks apart when probed with a fork. After a couple of hours, check the pork and add a little more water if necessary to keep it moist. Shred the pork with forks on a board or hot dish, discarding the rind and fat. Serve with a spoonful of the spicy cooking liquid on top.

**Nutritional facts**

192 cals, Protein 28g, Fats 5 g, Fiber 0.5 g, Carbs 3g

# 4.14 Sausages with Onion Gravy and Cauliflower Mash

On a low-carb diet, who'd have guessed you can use sausages and mash? You use cauliflower in our creamy mash,' which tastes just as fantastic. Freshly cooked vegetables such as wilted spinach, sliced cabbage, or beans should be added in large quantities.

Preparation time: 50 minutes

Cooking time: 1 hour

Serving: 4

**Ingredients**

- 2 tsp. olive or rapeseed oil
- 12 good-quality, high-meat sausages (375 gram pack)
- 1 medium onion, peeled and thinly sliced
- 300ml hot broth (½ pork or ½ chicken broth cube)
- 2 tbsp. reduced sugar tomato ketchup

- 2 tsp. corn flour

## For the cauliflower mash

- 1 medium cauliflower, trimmed, cut into small florets and stalk thinly sliced (700g prepared weight)

- 1 tablespoon olive oil

## Instructions

Take a medium saucepan, half-full it with water, and bring it to a boil to prepare the cauliflower mash. Return the pot to a boil with the cauliflower. Cook for 15–20 minutes, or until the vegetables are very soft. Return to the pan after draining. Add the olive oil, a pinch of sea salt, and a generous amount of powdered black pepper. Blend until smooth with a hand blending machine or in a food processor after cooling somewhat.

You can also take a potato peeler to peel the potatoes well. Warm over a low heat, stirring once in a while. Put the oil in a nonstick pan and gently cook the sausages for 5 minutes, flipping occasionally. Cook for a further 8 to 15 minutes, or until the sausages are fully cooked and the onion is very soft and browned.

Bring the stock and ketchup to a boil, then reduce to low heat. Mix the corn flour and one tablespoon cold water in a small dish, then stir into the pan. Season with freshly ground black pepper and cook, constantly stirring, for 1–2 minutes, or until thickened and glossy. Season with salt and pepper to taste. Top the cauliflower mash with the sausages and gravy and serve on four hot plates.

**Nutritional facts**

367 cals, Protein 19 g, Fats 25 g, Fiber 4.5 g, Carbs 15 g

## 4.15 Cheat's One-Pot Cassoulet

Beans, like lentils, are high in fiber and have even been shown to improve sleep quality. Serve with plenty of green leafy veggies, steaming hot.

Preparation time: 40 minutes

Cooking time: 1 hour

Serving: 4

**Ingredients**

- 1 tablespoon olive oil

- 6 spicy sausages (around 400g), such as Toulouse or spicy pork

- 1 large onion, peeled and thinly sliced

- 100 grams cubed smoked lardons, pancetta or bacon

- 400 grams can make haricot drained and rinsed

- 400 grams can chopped tomatoes

- 1 teaspoon dried mixed herbs

- Generous handful chopped fresh parsley, to serve

**Instructions**

In a wide-based, nonstick skillet or flame-proof casserole, heat the oil, then add the sausages and cook, frequently rotating, for about 5 minutes, or until lightly browned on all sides. Remove from the pan and place on a cutting board. Cook for 3–5 minutes, frequently turning, until the onion and pancetta are brown. Return the sausages to the pan, cut them in half, and add the beans, tomatoes, and herbs. 150ml water stirred in and brought to a slow simmer. Cook, stirring periodically, for 18–20 minutes, covered loosely. If the sauce is sticky too much, add a drop of water. To serve, season to taste with sea salt and plenty of black pepper, then toss in the parsley.

**Nutritional facts**

445 cals, Protein 30 g, Fats 26 g, Fiber 8 g, Carbs 19 g

## 4.16 Pan-Fried Pork with Apple and Leek

A delicious and substantial pork meal. And one that contains prebiotic fiber, which your gut microorganisms will like. Serve with a generous serving of freshly cooked leafy greens, courgette, or green beans on the side.

Preparation time: 50 minutes

Cooking time: 45 minutes

Serving: 2

## Ingredients

- 2 pork loin steaks (each around 135g)
- 1 tbsp. olive or rapeseed oil
- 1 small apple, quartered, cored and sliced
- 1 medium leek cut into roughly 1cm slices
- 200ml pork or chicken stock (made with ½ stock cube)
- 1 tsp. Dijon or wholegrain mustard
- 45g full-fat crème fraiche (around 3 tbsp)

## Instructions

Season each side of the pork with a pinch of sea salt and a generous amount of ground black pepper. Take a nonstick pan and warm the oil over medium heat and fry the pork for 3 to 8 minutes on both sides, or until lightly browned and cooked through, depending on thickness. If you overcook the pork, it will become tough.

Place on a platter that has been warmed. Cook for 2 minutes, or until the apple and leek are lightly browned and softened in the frying pan. Bring the broth and mustard to a boil, then reduce to low heat. Cook, constantly stirring, for 3 minutes, or until the leek is tender and the liquid has reduced by about two-thirds. Cook, constantly stirring, until the crème fraiche has melted and is boiling. Before serving, place the pork in the pan and warm it through for a minute or two.

## Nutritional facts

355 cals, Protein 32g, Fats 21 g, Fiber 3.5 g, Carbs 7 g

---

# 4.17 Peppered Pork Stir-Fry

A super-fast, super-delicious stir-fry.

Preparation time: 40 minutes

Cooking time: 45 minutes

Serving: 2

## Ingredients

- 250 grams pork tenderloin (fillet), sliced, cut in half lengthwise, then into 1cm slices
- 1 tablespoon coconut or rapeseed oil
- 320 to 350 grams pack mixed stir-fry vegetables
- 15 grams root ginger peeled and finely grated

## For the spicy sauce

- 1 teaspoon corn flour
- 1 tablespoon dark soy sauce
- 1 teaspoon honey
- ¼ to ½ teaspoon crushed chili flakes

## Instructions

Season the pork with a little bit of salt and plenty of freshly ground black pepper all over. Take a large nonstick frying pan or wok, heat the oil over medium-high heat. Stir in the pork for 3–4 minutes, tossing regularly, or until lightly browned and cooked through. Stir-fry the vegetables with the meat for 2–3 minutes. Cook for a few more seconds after adding the ginger. Combine the corn flour, soy sauce, honey, and chili in a separate bowl for the spicy sauce. Stir the veggies into the pan and toss everything together for 1–2 minutes, or until cooked and shiny. If desired, top with a bit of additional soy sauce.

## Nutritional facts

276 cals, Protein 29 g, FATs 11 g, Fiber 5g, Carbs 12.5 g

## 4.18 Parma Pork

A beautiful roast made with only three ingredients and less than ten minutes of prep time. It also reheats well for lunch or supper the next day. Serve with plenty of shredded kale, cabbage, or other greens that have been freshly cooked.

Preparation time: 1 hour

Cooking time: 1 hour

Serving: 3

## Ingredients

- 1-kilogram butternut

- 400-gram pork tenderloin (fillet) trimmed of fat and sinew

- 3 slices Parma ham or prosciutto

## Instructions

Preheat the oven to 200 °F and coat the baking tray with foil. Prick the whole, unpeeled squash with the tip of a knife 8–10 times on the baking tray. 1 hour in the oven

Wrap the pork in Parma ham or prosciutto in the meantime. Return the pork to the oven, along with the squash, for another 20 to 30minutes, or till the pork is cooked and the squash is soft. (You should be able to easily pierce the squash with a knife.) Place the pork on a heating platter and cover with foil to rest. Meanwhile, split the squash in half vertically, scoop out, and discard the seeds using a large spoon. Place the flesh in a basin after scooping it out of the skin. Season with salt and freshly ground black pepper, then mash thoroughly. Put the pork on a cutting wood board and slice thickly, saving the resting juices. Serve the mash on hot plates with the pork on top. To serve, drizzle with the juices.

## Nutritional facts

308 cals, Protein 35 g, Fats 7 g, Fiber 6 g, Carbs 23.5 g

## 4.19 Courgetti Spaghetti with Nuts, Spinach and Pancetta

A small amount of spaghetti adds texture to this delectable carbonara without adding too many calories. Serve with a salad — for added antioxidants, use radicchio or red chicory.

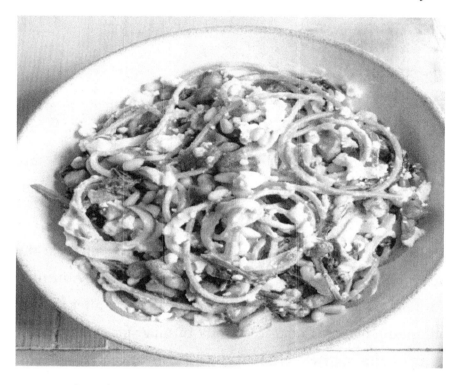

Preparation time: 45 minutes

Cooking time: 30 minutes

Serving: 2

**Ingredients**

- 80g dried whole wheat spaghetti

- 1 large courgette, trimmed and spiralized (20g pine nuts

- 50g cubed smoked lardons or pancetta (or diced bacon)

- 1 tbsp. olive oil

- 150g young spinach leaves

- 80g feta

## Instructions

Bring a big pot half-filled with water to a boil. Bring to a boil again and simmer for 10 to 15 minutes, until either the spaghetti is cooked. Add the spiralized courgette and mix rapidly to combine, then drain through a colander and run under cold water for a few seconds.

Meanwhile, in a nonstick saucepan with half the oil, toast the pine nuts and lardons for 2 to 3 minutes, frequently turning, until lightly browned. Return the pan to the heat after tipping out onto a platter. Cook, frequently turning, for 1–2 minutes, or until the spinach is tender, with the remaining oil and spinach. Sprinkle with salt and pepper and simmer till the two-thirds of the feta has melted, creating a creamy coating for the spinach.

Return the spaghetti and courgette to the pot, add the spinach and feta sauce, and mix thoroughly for 1– 2 minutes over medium heat, using two forks. Divide the feta between two shallow bowls, top with the pancetta and pine nuts, and crumble the remaining feta on top.

**Nutritional facts**

461 cals, Protein 21 g, Fats 27 g, Fiber 7 g, Carbs 29 g

## 4.20 Lamb Chops with Minted Peas and Feta

It is a quick, easy, and delicious supper. Serve with a green salad or wilted spinach (which is much better with a spoonful of olive oil or butter – adds 40 calories).

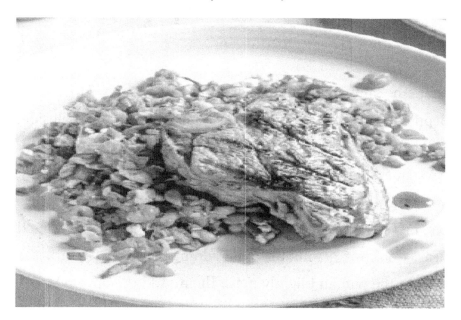

Preparation time: 2 hour

Cooking time: 1 hour 45 minutes

Serving: 2

## Ingredients

- 2 thick lamb loin chops around 175 grams or 4 lamb cutlets

- 1 teaspoon olive oil For the crushed peas and feta

- 200g frozen peas

- 1 tablespoon olive oil

- 15-gram pine nuts toasted

- 1 red chili finely diced

- 10 grams fresh mint leaves finely chopped

- 50 grams feta

## Instructions

Sauté the lamb on both sides with sea salt and powdered black pepper. Cook the chops for at least 3 to 7 minutes on each side, depending on thickness, or until done to taste, on a grill, barbeque, or frying pan over medium-high heat. In the end, switch to the fat side for 30 seconds. In the meantime, fill a pan halfway with water and bring to a boil to create the minted peas. Cook for 3 minutes after adding the peas. Return the peas to the pan and lightly mash them. Add the olive oil, pine nuts, and chili, then top with the mint and feta crumbles. Toss lightly with a generous amount of ground black pepper. To serve, divide the lamb and smashed peas between two plates.

## Nutritional facts

542 cals, Protein 47 g, Fats 33 g, Fiber 5 g, Carbs 12 g

# Chapter 5: Dinner

## 5.1 Lamb Saag

A simple toss-it-all-in-the-oven curry that you can put in the oven and forget about. For the most significant results, use a high-quality curry paste. Serve with cucumber and onion salad and cauliflower rice.

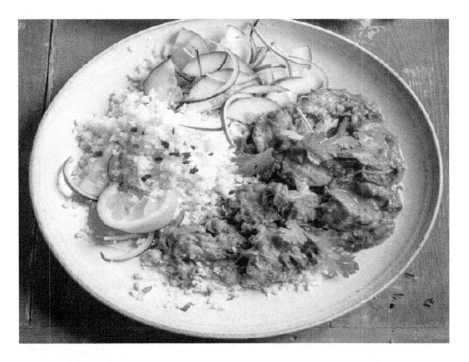

Preparation time: 1 hour

Cooking time: 4 hours

Serving: 4

**Ingredients**

- 1 tablespoon coconut or rapeseed oil

- 1 medium onion, peeled and finely sliced

- 500 grams lamb neck fillets, trimmed and cut into roughly 3–4cm chunks

- 60g (around 4 tbsp.) medium Indian curry paste, such as rogan josh or tikka masala

- 50 grams dried red split lentils

- 200 grams frozen spinach

## Instructions

Preheat the oven to 180 °C. Heat the oil in a flame-safe pan and gently sauté the onion for 5 minutes, or till it gets softened and golden brown. Season the lamb chunks with sea salt and ground black pepper and cook for 3 minutes, flipping frequently, or until browned on all sides. Cook for 1 minute with the lamb and onion after adding the curry paste. Stir in 500ml water with the lentils and spinach. Bring to a boil, then cover and bake for 1–4 hours, or until the lamb is tender and the sauce has thickened.

## Nutritional facts

361 cals, Protein 29 g, Fats 21.5g, Fiber 3.5 g, Carbs 10.5 g

## 5.2 Spiced Lamb and Minted Yogurt

Spice-crusted lamb with colorful Mediterranean veggies is a classic pairing.

Preparation time: 1 hour

Cooking time: 2 hours

Serving: 2

## Ingredients

- ½ teaspoon ground cumin

- ½ teaspoon ground coriander

- 2 lean boneless lamb leg steaks (each around 100g)

- 2 tablespoon olive oil

- 1 medium onion skinned cut into 12 small portions

- 1 pepper cut into roughly 3cm portions

- 1 medium courgette halved lengthwise cut into roughly 1.5cm slices

- For the minted yogurt sauce

- 100g full-Fats live Greek yoghurt

- ½ small garlic clove, peeled and crushed

- 2 tablespoon finely chopped fresh mint leaves

## Instructions

Combine the cumin, coriander, a pinch of sea salt, and plenty of ground black pepper on a plate. Coat both sides of the lamb steaks with the spice mixture and set aside. Combine the yogurt, garlic, and mint in a small dish, then add just enough cold water to produce a drizzling consistency. Take a nonstick frying pan, heat 1 tablespoon of the oil and gently cook the onion, pepper,

and courgette for 4–5 minutes, stirring frequently. Push the veggies to one side of the pan, add the remaining 1 tablespoon oil, and cook the steaks for at least 3 to 4 minutes on each side, or until done to your liking, over medium heat. (To avoid burning the vegetables, turn them occasionally while the lamb is cooking.) Allow for 5 minutes of resting time before dividing between two dishes and drizzle with yogurt sauce.

**Nutritional facts**

377 cals, Protein 25 g, Fats 24.5 g, Fiber 4 g, Carbs 12 g

## 5.3 Meatballs in Tomato Sauce

You can make this dish with the classic Mediterranean flavors suggested here or give it a more exotic Moroccan taste. Serve with a large helping of lightly cooked courgette and

A leafy salad.

Preparation time: 45 minutes

Cooking time: 50 minutes

Serving: 4

## Ingredients

- 300 grams small good-quality beef meatballs (around 20)

- 1 tablespoon olive oil

- 1 medium onion, peeled and finely chopped

- 2 garlic cloves, peeled and crushed

- 400g can chopped tomatoes

- 1 teaspoon dried oregano

- ¼–½ teaspoon crushed dried chili flakes (optional)

## Instructions

Preheat the oven to 200 °C. Heat the oil in a flame-safe pan and gently sauté the onion for 5 minutes, or till it gets softened and golden brown. Cook the meatballs for 10 minutes on a baking sheet. Meanwhile, in a large nonstick frying pan, heat the oil and gently cook the onion for 5 minutes, or till it gets soft and golden browned, stirring frequently. Cook for a few seconds longer, stirring constantly. Bring the tomatoes, 200ml water, oregano, and chili, if using, to a gentle simmer in the pan. Cook for 5 minutes, stirring occasionally. Place the meatballs in the tomato sauce when they have been removed from the oven. Cook for another 5 minutes, or until the meatballs are thoroughly cooked, seasoning with sea salt and ground black pepper. If the sauce is dense too much, add a drop of water to thin it down.

**Nutritional facts**

272 cals, Protein 16 g, Fats 20 g, Fiber 2 g, Carbs 7 g

## 5.4 Simple Steak and Salad

A delicious steak with a colorfully tossed salad on a fast day is a terrific, simple, low-carb combination that delivers a good Protein boost.

Preparation time: 30 minutes

Cooking time: 25 minutes

Serving: 2

**Ingredients**

- 225 grams lean sirloin beef steak, cut in half

- 1 tablespoon olive oil

- 150 grams button chestnut mushrooms sliced if large

## For the salad

- 100g mixed leaves

- ½ yellow pepper, deseeded and sliced

- 10 cherry tomatoes, halved

- 1/3 cucumber (around 135g), sliced

- 2 spring onions, trimmed and finely sliced

## For the balsamic dressing

- 2 tablespoon extra-virgin olive oil

- 2 teaspoon balsamic vinegar

## Instructions

To make the salad, combine all of the ingredients in a large mixing basin. Season the beef with sea salt and a generous amount of ground black pepper all over.

Take a large nonstick frying pan, heat the oil over medium-high heat and cook the steaks for a minimum of 5 minutes on both sides, or until done to your liking. Place the steaks on two hot plates to rest for a few minutes. Cook, frequently stirring, for 2 to 4 minutes, or until the mushrooms are browned. On top of the steaks, spoon the sauce. Toss the salad with a slight drizzle of oil and vinegar. Serve with the steak and mushrooms on the side.

### Nutritional facts

346 cals, Protein 30 g, Fats 22 g, Fiber 3 g, CARBS 5 g

## 5.5 Pie with Swede Mash

A low-carb version of a family favorite. You may consume leftovers the following day or freeze them. Serve with a slew of freshly cooked green vegetables on the side.

Preparation time: 30 minutes

Cooking time: 45 minutes

Serving: 5

## Ingredients

- 2 tablespoon olive oil

- 500 grams lean minced beef (around 10% Protein)

- 1 medium onion, peeled and finely chopped

- 200 grams carrots (around 2 medium), trimmed and cut into roughly 1cm chunks

- 1 beef stock cube

- 2 tablespoon tomato purée

- 1 tablespoon Worcestershire sauce

- 1 teaspoon dried mixed herbs

- 1.2kg swede (around 1 large or 2 small), peeled and cut into roughly 3cm chunks

- 150 grams frozen peas

## Instructions

Take a large nonstick saucepan, heat the oil and cook the mince, onion, and carrots for 6 to 10 minutes, or until the mince is browned and the onions have softened. Over the mince, crumble the stock cube and add 700ml water, the tomato purée, Worcestershire sauce, and herbs. Season generously with sea salt and powdered black pepper and bring to a simmer. Cook, stirring regularly and adding a little more water if necessary, for about 25 minutes, covered loosely. The tender and saucy mince should be used.

Preheat the oven to 220°C. Meanwhile, throw the swede in a large pot and cover it with cold water to prepare the swede mash. Bring to a boil, covered with a cap. Cook for 20 minutes, or until the potatoes are tender. Drain the swede in a sieve, then return to the pan and mash till smooth as possible with a potato masher. Sprinkle the salt and black pepper.

Cook for 1 minute, stirring regularly, after adding the frozen peas to the mince. Pour into a 2-liter shallow ovenproof dish with care. Bake for 15 to 25minutes, or till the swede is tipped with brown and the filling is bubbling, or until the swede is tipped with brown and the filling is bubbling. (Unlike mashed potatoes, it will not get golden.)

**Nutritional facts**

354 cals, Protein 27 g, Fats 16 g, Fiber 10 g, Carbs 21 g

## 5.6 Beef Stroganoff

This flavorful, filling beef stew incorporates a plethora of beautiful mushrooms, which offer extra flavor and texture while adding very few calories. Serve with a mixed side salad and cauliflower rice or courgette.

Preparation time: 35 minutes

Cooking time: 50 minutes

Serving: 2

## Ingredients

- 250 grams sirloin steak

- 2 tablespoon olive oil

- 1 medium onion, peeled and thinly sliced

- 150 grams button chestnut mushrooms, sliced

- 1 teaspoon paprika (not smoked)

- 175ml beef stock (made with ½ beef stock cube)

- 2 teaspoon corn flour

- 30 grams (around 2 tablespoon) full-Protein crème fraiche

- Chopped fresh parsley, to serve

## Instructions

Remove any excess Protein from the steak and cut it into long, thin strips that are no more than 1cm broad on a slight diagonal. Season with salt and ground black pepper.

Take a nonstick frying pan, heat 1 tablespoon of the oil over medium-high heat. Cook for 2–3 minutes, or until the steak is browned but not cooked through. Return the pan to heat and remove the steak to a platter.

Cook for 4–5 minutes, or until the onions are softened and lightly browned, using the remaining oil in the pan is onion and mushrooms.

Cook for a few more seconds after adding the paprika.

Bring the broth to a low fire in the pan. Cook, frequently stirring, for 2 minutes.

Mix the corn flour and 1 tablespoon fresh water in a small dish, then stir into the pan. Put the steak in the pan with the crème fraiche. Warm the meat in the sauce for 1–2 minutes, stirring frequently and adding a splash of water if necessary. To serve, garnish with chopped fresh parsley.

**Nutritional facts**

392 cals, Protein 33 g, Fats 23.5g, Fiber 3 g, Carbs 11 g

## 5.7 Classic Burger with Celeriac Chips

Adding grated carrot to burgers adds moisture and fiber to the dish. You can still eat your chips with this low-carb dish. With a large mixed salad, serve the burgers.

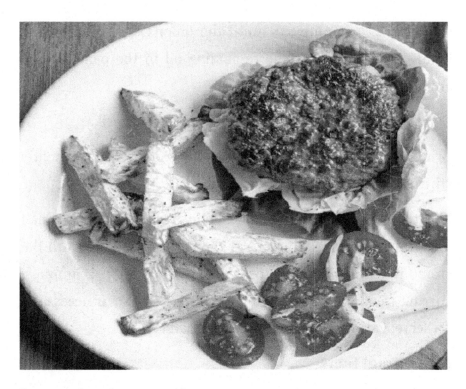

Preparation time: 30 minutes

Cooking time: 30 minutes

Serving: 4

**Ingredients**

- ½ onion peeled and coarsely grated

- 1 garlic clove, peeled and finely grated

- 100 grams carrot (around 1 medium), trimmed and finely grated

- 400 grams lean minced beef around 10% Protein

- ½ teaspoon flaked sea salt

- ½ teaspoon dried mixed herbs

- For the celeriac chips

- 750 grams celeriac peeled around 600 grams peeled weight

- 1 tablespoon rapeseed oil

## Instructions

Preheat the oven to 220 °C.

To create the celeriac chips:

1. Cut the celeriac into 1.5cm slices and then into chips using a sharp knife.

2. Combine with the oil, a pinch of sea salt, and a generous amount of ground black pepper in a mixing bowl.

3. Toss everything together thoroughly.

4. Bake for 20 minutes after scattering onto a baking tray.

5. Return to the oven for another 5–10 minutes, or until the chips are soft and gently browned.

Make the burgers in the meantime. Take a mixing bowl, add the onion, garlic, carrot, minced, salt, and dried mixed herbs, season with black pepper, and mix well with your hands.

Make four balls out of the mixture and flatten them into burger shapes. Because they will shrink as they cook, make them a little flatter than you think they should be.

Cook the burgers without any additional grease in a large nonstick frying pan over medium heat for 10 minutes, or till it becomes lightly browned and cooked through, rotating periodically. With a spatula, press the burgers now and then to ensure equal cooking. Serve the chips on four hot plates with a burger on the side.

**Nutritional facts**

259 cals, Protein 24 g, Fats 13.5 g, Fiber 8 g, Carbs 6 g

## 5.8 Beef Rending

This recipe is a simplified version of a Malaysian staple, yet it is wonderfully tasty and filling. Serve with steaming spring greens, broccoli with long stems, or pak choi.

Preparation time: 40 minutes

Cooking time: 1 hour

Serving: 4

**Ingredients**

- 600-gram beef braising steak cut into roughly 4cm pieces
- 6 garlic cloves, peeled
- 50 grams fresh ginger roughly chopped
- 2 medium red onions, peeled and quartered
- 1 teaspoon crushed dried chili flakes

- 2 tablespoon coconut or rapeseed oil

- 400ml can coconut milk

- 3 tablespoon soya sauce

- 1 beef stock cube

- ½ teaspoon cinnamon

- 2 stalks lemongrass, trimmed (optional)

- lime wedges, to serve

**Instructions**

Preheat the oven to 170 °C. Sea salt and black pepper should be used to season the beef.

Pulse the garlic, ginger, onions, and chili flakes until very finely chopped in a food processor. Take a large nonstick frying pan, heat 1 tablespoon of the oil over high heat. Transfer the meat to a flame-proof casserole dish in two batches and fry until lightly browned on all sides. Cook the garlic and onion combined in the same pan with the remaining oil for 5 minutes, stirring often.

Stir in the coconut milk, soya sauce, and 200ml water to the casserole with the beef. In a small bowl, crumble the stock cube and stir in the cinnamon. If using lemongrass, snap each stalk twice without entirely separating the pieces or smash with a rolling pin before adding to the curry (this will release the flavor). Bring to a low simmer, stirring constantly. Cook for

234–314 hours in the oven, covered, or until the beef is meltingly soft.

**Nutritional facts**

482 cals, Protein 36 g, Fats 31.5 g, Fiber 2.5 g, Carbs 12.5 g

## 5.9 Speedy Pizza

The perfect wholegrain pizza is also the quickest to make! Serve with a large mixed salad as a side dish.

Preparation time: 20 minutes

Cooking time: 20 minutes

Serving: 2

**Ingredients**

- 227 grams can chopped tomatoes (400g can)

- 1 tablespoon tomato sauce

- ½ teaspoon dried oregano roughly chopped fresh oregano leaves

- 1 whole meal pitta bread around 58 grams

- 2 roasted red peppers around 40 grams washed and sliced

- 2 chestnut mushrooms around 45 grams very finely sliced

- 35 grams ready-grated mozzarella

- 1 tablespoon extra-virgin olive oil

## Instructions

Preheat the grill to medium-high temperature. To make the pizza topping, strain the tomatoes over a strainer to eliminate extra liquid. (You don't have to press it.) Toss the tomato pulp with the tomato purée and oregano in a mixing dish. Season with a pinch of salt and a generous amount of freshly ground black pepper.

Place the pita bread on a board and lightly toast it to warm it up, then gently cut it in half horizontally with a bread knife and separate the two oval pieces.

Top with the peppers, mushrooms, and mozzarella after spreading the tomato sauce on the pita halves. Grilled for 4 to 5 minutes, or till the cheese has melted and the tomato topping, mushrooms, and peppers are heated.

## Nutritional facts

221cals, Protein 9 g, Fats 11.5 g, Fiber 4.5 g, Carbs 18.5 g

## 5.10 Smoked Haddock with Lentils

A simple one-pan recipe in which the fish's slightly Smokey, salty flavor stands out and complements the earthiness of the lentils. Serve with a considerable amount of sautéed leafy greens on the side.

Preparation time: 25 minutes

Cooking time: 30 minutes

Serving: 2

**Ingredients**

- 2 tablespoon olive oil
- ½ medium onion, peeled and finely chopped
- 1 celery stick, trimmed and finely sliced
- 1 medium carrot, trimmed, halved lengthways and diagonally sliced
- 1 rosemary sprig or ¼ teaspoon dried rosemary
- 1 garlic clove very finely sliced
- 250 grams sachet ready-cooked lentils
- 200ml vegetable stock (made with ½ stock cube)
- 140 grams smoked haddock or cod fillets, skinned
- A small handful of parsley leaves

**Instructions**

In a nonstick frying pan or a wide-based saucepan, heat the oil over low heat. Cook for 5 minutes, or till the onion becomes soft and carrots are tender but not browned.

Cook for a few seconds more, constantly stirring, after adding the rosemary and garlic. Pour the stock over the lentils in the pan. Bring to a moderate simmer before adding the fish fillets.

Season with freshly ground black pepper and, if desired, chopped parsley.

Cook the fish for about 8 minutes, or until it begins to flake when probed with a knife, covered with a lid (or a heatproof plate). Top the lentils with the fish and serve on two warmed plates or bowls.

**Nutritional facts**

434 cals, Protein 42 g, Fats 14 g, Fiber 11 g, Carbs 29 g

## 5.11 Pan-Fried Fish with Lemon and Parsley

This is an excellent one-person supper, but it can easily be doubled. Cook your veggies or make a salad before starting to fry the fish, as it just takes 5 minutes. If plaice isn't your thing, sea bass or sea bream are suitable substitutes.

Preparation time: 30 minutes

Cooking time: 20 minutes

Serving: 1

**Ingredients**

- 1 plaice fillet (around 175g), or other white fish fillet, thawed if frozen

- 15 gram butter

- 1 tablespoon extra-virgin olive oil

- 1 tablespoon fresh lemon juice

- Small bunch fresh parsley, leaves finely chopped (around 2 tbsp.)

## Instructions

Season the skinless side of the fish with salt and black pepper. Take a nonstick frying pan, melt the butter with the oil over medium heat. Cook for 3 minutes with the place skin-side down. Turn carefully and cook for another 1–2 minutes on the other side, depending on the thickness of the fillet. (If you choose, you can carefully peel off the skin.) With a fish slice or spatula, lift the plaice onto a hot plate, skin side down. Return the pan to heat, add the lemon juice and parsley, and frequently whisk for a few seconds. To serve, pour the buttery liquids over the fish.

## Nutritional facts

368cals, Protein 33 g, Fats 26 g, Fiber 0.5 g, Carbs 0.5 g

## 5.12 Crunchy Fish Bites

Delicious chunks of white fish with a golden polenta and crushed almonds coating. You won't miss the starchy, breaded, or battered varieties once you've tried them. Serve with freshly cooked greens or a large mixed salad.

Preparation time: 25 minutes

Cooking time: 30 minutes

Serving: 2

**Ingredients**

- 1 medium egg

- 40 grams quick-cook polenta (fine cornmeal)

- 20 grams ground almonds

- 275 grams thick skinless white fish fillet (such as cod, haddock or Pollock), cut into roughly 3cm chunks

- 2 tablespoon olive or rapeseed oil

- Lemon wedges, to serve

**Instructions**

Take a small mixing bowl, whisk together the egg and season with salt and pepper.

In a separate bowl, combine the polenta and almonds. Season with black pepper and sea salt. Turn the pieces of fish in the beaten egg one at a time until thoroughly coated, then toss in the polenta mixture. Place on a platter and set away. Place a big nonstick frying pan over medium heat and pour in the oil. Fry the fish bites for 5–7 minutes, depending on thickness, until cooked through, golden brown, and crisp on all sides, flipping occasionally. Lemon is also served on the side for squeezing.

**Nutritional facts**

383 cals, Protein 33 g, Fats 21 g, Fiber 0.6 g, Carbs 15 g

## 5.13 Mediterranean Fish Bake

In this simple tray bake, roasted Mediterranean-style vegetables pair beautifully with the fish. Serve with a salad or slender green beans as a side dish.

Preparation time: 20 minutes

Cooking time: 45 minutes

Serving: 2

**Ingredients**

- 1 medium red onion cut into 12 parts
- 1 red pepper cut into roughly 2cm chunks
- 1 courgette halved lengthways and cut into roughly 2cm chunks

- 2 medium tomatoes, quartered

- 1½ tablespoon olive oil

- 100 grams sea bass or sea bream fillets

- 40 grams pitted black olives (preferably Kalamata), drained

- Juice ½ large lemon, plus extra wedges to serve

## Instructions

Preheat the oven to 200 °C. Scatter the onion, pepper, courgette and tomato quarters on a large baking stray. Toss everything together with 1 tablespoon of oil drizzled on top. Roast for 20

minutes, seasoning with sea salt and freshly ground black pepper. Retrieve the dish from the oven and season the fish with pepper before placing it skin-side downwards amongst some vegetables. Sprinkle the olives on topping after squeezing the lemon zest over the top.

Return the dish to the oven there for another approximately 10 min, until either the vegetables are supple or the salmon is cooked through. Serve the fish and veggies on two hot plates with the remaining oil drizzled on top and lemon wedges on the side.

## Nutritional facts

384 cals, Protein 24 g, Fats 23.5 g, Fiber 0 g, Carbs 15 g

# 5.14 Swedish Spicy Carrot with Cod

On a silky carrot purée, juicy fish steaks are served. Heaven. A memorable supper inspired this recipe in Stockholm following a 5:2 conference. Half a plate of cooked green vegetables, such as long-stemmed broccoli, spring greens, or kale, should be served alongside.

Preparation time: 30minutes

Cooking time: 35 minutes

Serving: 2

## Ingredients

- 2 large carrots (around 300 grams), trimmed and thickly sliced

- 1 garlic clove, peeled

- 15 grams fresh root ginger, peeled

- 15 grams butter

- ½ tablespoon fresh lemon juice

- 150 grams thick, skinless cod fillets (or other white fish)

- 1 tablespoon olive oil

- Good pinch dried chili flakes

## Instructions

Take a medium saucepan, add the carrots, garlic, and ginger with water. Bring to a boil, then reduce to low heat and cook for 15 minutes, or until the vegetables are tender.

Remove the carrot, garlic, and ginger from the pan, scoop out, set aside a ladleful of water (about 100ml), and drain. Return the potatoes to the pan with 3 tablespoons of the cooking liquid, the butter, and the lemon juice. Using a stick blender, blitz the carrots until they're a smooth, creamy purée, applying a little more boiling water if required. To taste, stir with salt and black pepper. Take it out of the equation.

Coat the fish fillets on both sides with salt and black pepper. Heat the oil in a greased frying pan over medium heat. After adding the fish, cook for 4 minutes. Turn the fish over, sprinkle with a few chili flakes, and cook for 3–5 minutes more, depending on the thickness of each fillet. When the cod begins to flake into huge chunks, it is ready. Place the purée on two warmed plates and top with the fish.

**Nutritional facts**

279cals, Protein 27.5 g, Fats 13.5 g, Fiber 5 g, Carbs 9 g

## 5.15 Ginger and Chili Baked Fish

A simple baked fish recipe that serves one person but may easily be duplicated for additional servings. Although we used cod, any thick white fish will suffice. Half the plate should be filled with long-stemmed broccoli, mange tout, or stir-fried veggies.

Preparation time: 30 minutes

Cooking time: 40 minutes

Serving: 1

**Ingredients**

- 2 teaspoon olive oil

- 175 grams thick white fish fillet, such as cod (preferably skinned)

- 1 garlic clove, peeled and thinly sliced

- 15 grams stem ginger (around ½ ball), drained and cut into thin matchsticks

- 1 spring onion, trimmed and diagonally sliced

- 1 red bird's eye chili, thinly sliced, or ¼ tsp crushed dried chili flakes

- Juice ½ small lime, plus extra wedges to serve

- Handful fresh coriander leaves

## Instructions

Preheat the oven to 200 °C. Drizzle the oil over a rectangle of kitchen foil on a baking tray.

Place the fish on half of the foil, skin side down, with enough foil to cover it. Garlic, ginger, spring onion, and chili are sprinkled over the fish, and lime juice is squeezed over it. Toss the fish with salt and black pepper prior to actually folding the foil over it and rolling up the edges to seal it within. Because steam is required to cook the fish, make sure the package isn't too tight.

Oven preheated to 350°F and bake the fish for approximately 20 minutes, or until a fork pierces the fish and it flakes into big pieces.

Using a fish slice or spatula, carefully open the foil bundle and lift the fish onto a warming platter. Serve the fish with the cooking fluids, lots of fresh coriander, and lime wedges on the side.

**Nutritional facts**

233 cals, Protein 31 g, Fats 7 g, Fiber 0.7 g, Carbs 11 g

## 5.16 Stir-Fry Tuna with Hoisin Sauce

After a long day, this simple tuna dish is the ideal lunch. Ready-to-use stir-fry veggie packs save time and are readily available. Alternatively, you can create your mix with any fresh, crisp vegetables. And don't sweat the slight differences in the calorie count of the stir-fried vegetables; simply enjoy them!

Preparation time: 35 minutes

Cooking time: 50 minutes

Serving: 1

**Ingredients**

- 110 grams fresh tuna steak, cut into roughly 3cm chunks

- 1 tablespoon coconut or rapeseed oil

- 300–350 grams pack stir-fry vegetables

- 2 tablespoon ready-made hoisin sauce

- Pinch crushed dried chili

## Instructions

Sprinkle the tuna with salt and black pepper on all sides. Heat the oil in a big nonstick frying pan or wok over high heat and stir fry the tuna and veggies for 3–4 minutes, or until the tuna is gently browned, or according to the package directions. Drizzle the hoisin sauce over the fish and veggies and toss for another 20– 30 seconds. If using, top with the chili flakes and serve right away.

## Nutritional facts

328 cals, Protein 31.5 g, Fats 13 g, Fiber 9 g, Carbs 16.5 g

## 5.17 Leek and Salmon Quiche in a Dish

By omitting the pastry crust, this simple salmon quiche is substantially reduced in calories and carbohydrates. Serve warm with a large green and red leaf salad, or cold as a high-Protein, nutritious addition to a packed lunch.

Preparation time:

Cooking time:

Serving: 2

## Ingredients

- 1 tablespoon olive oil, plus extra for greasing

- 1 medium leek, trimmed and thinly sliced (around 100g prepared weight)

- 1 garlic clove, peeled and crushed

- Generous handful of young spinach leaves (around 50g)

- 100 grams cooked salmon fillet, skinned

- 4 large eggs

- ½ tablespoon Fresh thyme leaves or ½ tsp. dried thyme

- 45 grams full-Protein crème fraiche

- 15 grams Parmesan, medium grated

**Instructions**

Preheat the oven to 190 °C. Oil a small ovenproof baking dish or two small dishes to hold roughly 900ml of liquid. Take a nonstick frying pan, boil the oil over medium heat. Add the \sleek and gently cook for 3 minutes, or until softened but not browned. Simmer, constantly whisking, for about 2 minutes until either the spinach has wilted and softened, adding the garlic and spinach a handful at a time.

Place the spinach in a sieve and squeeze the excess liquid out with the back of a spoon. Place the leeks and spinach in the greased dish or divide among the plates.

Flake the salmon into chunky pieces and combine with the leeks and spinach in the bottom of the plate, spreading loosely. Take a small bowl, whisk together the eggs, thyme, and crème fraiche. Stir in 2 tablespoons of Parmesan, season with salt and plenty of ground black pepper. Pour down the egg mixture over the fish and vegetables gently. Bake for 25 minutes (15–20 minutes if using two plates), or until slightly puffed up, golden brown, and just set.

**Nutritional facts**

507 cals, Protein 34.5 g, Fats 39.5 g, Fiber 2 g, Carbs 2.5 g

# 5.17 Sesame Salmon with Broccoli and Tomatoes

This dish is delicious hot for supper or cold for a quick lunch. If salmon isn't your thing, any other hefty fish fillet will suffice.

Preparation time: 30 minutes

Cooking time: 25 minutes

Serving: 2

**Ingredients**

- 2 teaspoons rapeseed oil

- 2 pieces of salmon fillets (125 grams each)

- 6 spring onions, trimmed and each cut into 3 pieces

- 12 cherry tomatoes

- 200g long-stemmed broccoli, trimmed

- 1 tablespoon soya sauce

- 1 teaspoon Sesame oil

- ½ teaspoon crushed dried chili flakes

- 1 teaspoon sesame seeds

## Instructions

Preheat the oven to 200 °C. Drizzle the oil over a baking tray. Place the salmon fillets down in the tray, along with the spring onions and tomatoes, and season generously with ground black pepper. Heated the oven to 350°F and bake for 8 minutes. In the meantime, fill a pan halfway with water and bring to a boil. Return the pot to a boil with the broccoli. Drain after 4 minutes of cooking. Place the broccoli on the baking tray after removing it from the oven. Soya sauce and sesame oil should be drizzled over the fish. Revert the salmon to the oven for the next 3 to 4 minutes, or until just done, then sprinkle with the chili powder and sesame seeds. Split it up between two heated plates to serve.

## Nutritional facts

403 cals, Protein 31.5 g, Fats 26 g, Fiber 6 g, Carbs 9 g

## 5.18 Thai Curry with Prawns

Creamy curry with Thai flavors that are incredibly filling. It's also super-quick and straightforward.

Preparation time: 20 minutes

Cooking time: 30 minutes

Serving: 2

## Ingredients

- 1 tablespoon coconut oil

- 1 red pepper cut into roughly 2cm chunks

- 4 spring onions thickly sliced

- 20 grams root ginger, peeled and finely grated

- 3 tablespoon Thai red or green curry paste

- ½ Can use coconut milk about 400ml

- 100g mange tout or sugar snap peas, halved

- 1 red chili, finely sliced, or ½ teaspoon dried chili

- 200 grams large cooked, peeled prawns, thawed if frozen

## Instructions

Take a large nonstick frying pan, heat the oil over medium-high heat and stir-fry the pepper for 2 minutes. Cook for another minute, constantly stirring, after adding the spring onions, ginger, and curry paste. Fill the pan halfway with coconut milk and bring to a medium simmer. If using, add the mange tout or sugar snap peas, as well as the chili. Return to low heat and cook for another 2 minutes, stirring occasionally.

Heat for 1–2 minutes, or until prawns are heated. If the sauce becomes thick too, add a drop of water. Serve with cauliflower rice that has just been cooked.

**Nutritional facts**

376 cals, Protein 18 g, Fats 27 g, Fiber 5 g, Carbs 13.5 g

## 5.19 Mussels with Creamy Tarragon Sauce

Mussels are a delicious, inexpensive, low-calorie, high-Protein entrée. Don't be put off if you've never cooked mussels before; they're really simple to prepare, and the quality of farmed mussels in the UK is excellent. Serve with a 50g sourdough or wholegrain bread slice (119cals).

Preparation time: 20 minutes

Cooking time: 25 minutes

Serving: 2

**Ingredients**

- 1kg fresh, live mussels

- 1 tablespoon olive oil

- 1 medium leek, trimmed and thinly sliced (around 100 grams prepared weight)

- 2 garlic cloves, peeled and thinly sliced

- 100ml dry white wine

- 75g full-Protein crème fraiche

- 3–4 fresh tarragon stalks (around 5 grams), leaves picked and roughly chopped/1 tsp. dried tarragon

## Instructions

Remove the 'beards' by dumping the mussels into the sink and scrubbing them thoroughly under cold running water. Mussels with fractured shells or those that do not close when pounded on the sink's side should be discarded. Drain the ones that are good in a colander.

In a deep, lidded, wide-based saucepan or shallow casserole, heat the oil over low heat. Gently sauté the leek and garlic for 2–3 minutes, or until softened but not browned.

Season generously with salt and pepper after adding the white wine, crème fraiche, and tarragon. Bring the wine to a simmer by increasing the heat under the pan.

Cook for about 4 minutes, or until most of the mussels have steamed open, after stirring in the mussels and covering closely with a lid. Stir thoroughly, then cover and cook for another 1–2 minutes, or until the rest of the vegetables are done.

Remove any mussels that haven't opened, divide the mussels between two bowls, and pour the tarragon broth over the top.

## Nutritional facts

381 cals, Protein 27 g, Fats 24 g, Fiber 2.5 g, Carbs 4 g

# 5.20 Prawn Nasi Goreng

Instead of basmati rice, cauliflower 'rice' is used in this quick, low-carb variation. Prepare everything before you begin cooking because it will just take a few minutes.

Preparation time: 20 minutes

Cooking time: 35 minutes

Serving: 2

## Ingredients

- 2 tablespoon coconut or rapeseed oil

- 1 medium onion, peeled and diced

- 1 red pepper cut into roughly 2cm chunks

- ½ small Savoy cabbage leaves thinly sliced (about 275 grams prepared weight)

- 2 garlic cloves, peeled and thinly sliced

- 20 grams root ginger, peeled and finely grated

- ½–1 teaspoon crushed dried chili flakes (to taste)

- 200g cauliflower rice (see tip)

- 2 tablespoon soya sauce

- 150 grams cooked peeled prawns, thawed if frozen

- Generous handful fresh coriander leaves roughly chopped (optional)

- 20 grams roasted peanuts, roughly chopped

**Instructions**

Take a large nonstick frying pan or wok, heat the oil over medium-high heat. 2–3 minutes, stirring constantly, stir-fry the onion, red pepper, and cabbage.

Stir in the garlic, ginger, chili, and cauliflower rice for another 2–3 minutes, or until the cauliflower is heated through.

Cook for another 1–2 minutes, swirling and tossing until the prawns are heated, before adding the soy sauce, prawns, and half of the coriander, if using. To taste:

1.  Add extra soy sauce.

2.  Top with the chopped nuts and the leftover coriander, if using, and divide between two bowls.

**Nutritional facts**

354 cals, Proteins 17 g, Fats 10g, Carbs 23 g, Fiber 3.5 g

# 5.21 Baked Salmon with Pea and Broccoli Mash

This recipe takes not more than 15 minutes to prepare.

Preparation time: 30 minutes

Cooking time: 35 minutes

Serving: 2

## Ingredients

- 15 grams butter, plus extra for greasing

- 225 grams fresh salmon fillets

- 150 grams frozen peas

- 150 grams broccoli cut into small florets and stalks thinly sliced

- 1 tablespoon finely chopped fresh mint (optional)

- Lemon wedges, to serve

## Instructions

Preheat the oven to 200 °C. Using foil, line a small baking pan and lightly coat it with butter.

Season the salmon with a bit of salt and some ground black pepper and place it skin-side down on the foil. Depending on thickness, bake for 10–12 minutes. On the other hand, half-fill a pan with water and boil to prepare the pea and broccoli mash. Return the pot to a boil with the peas and broccoli. Cook, occasionally stirring, for 5 minutes, or until the broccoli is cooked. Wash the veggies and return them to the pan with a tiny ladleful of the cooking water (about 75ml).

Stir with a stick blender until almost smooth, adding the butter, mint if using, and 3 tablespoons of the conserved cooking water. Season to taste, and loosen with a splash of water if necessary. Split the mash among two heated plates and top with the seared

salmon, which you can simply break open from the foil and discard. Serve with a lemon wedge. Serve with a wedge of lemon.

**Nutritional facts**

440 cals, Proteins 27 g, Fats 7 g, Carbs 11 g, Fiber 2.5 g

# Chapter 6: Salads

## 6.1 Quinoa, Broccoli and Asparagus Salad

A hearty salad with a beautiful lemony dressing. It's also delicious with grilled meat or fish. Extra leaves or salad parts, such as rockets, can be added.

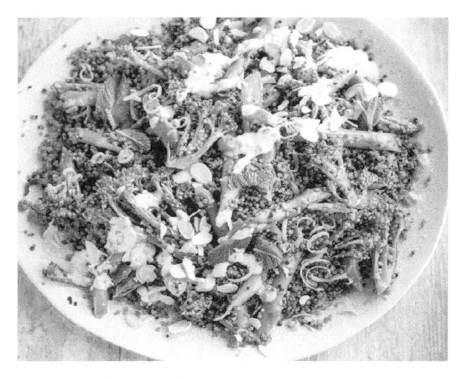

Preparation time: 10 minutes

Cooking time: 18 minutes

Serving: 2

**Ingredients**

- 100 grams quinoa a mixture of white, red and black

- 100 grams asparagus, trimmed and each stem cut into three

- 25 grams toasted flaked almonds

- 100 grams long-stemmed broccoli (trimmed and each stem cut into three)

## For the minted Yogurt dressing

- 50g full-fat live Greek yogurt

- 1 tablespoon extra-virgin olive oil

- 1 tablespoon finely chopped fresh mint

- Finely grated zest and juice ½ lemon

- Pinch ground cumin

## Instructions

Pour a pot halfway with water and bring to a boil. Cook, stirring periodically, for 12–15 minutes, or until quinoa is just tender. When the quinoa is cooked, the shaped husks will begin to float to the surface. Rinse the quinoa thoroughly in a colander under cold running water. Drain the quinoa thoroughly again, pushing the quinoa in the sieve with the back of a spoon to get as much water as possible.

In the meantime, heat a second pot of water and cook the broccoli and asparagus for 3 minutes. Rinse the asparagus and broccoli under cold running water after draining them. To prepare the filling, toss together all ingredients in a small mixing bowl with only enough icy water to make it pourable. Toss with salt and black pepper to taste. Take a large mixing bowl, combine the quinoa, asparagus, broccoli, and flaked almonds. Toss with black pepper and salt to taste. Splash the dressing over the salad before serving.

**Nutritional facts**

362 cals, Protein 15 g, Fats 18 g, Fiber 7 g, Carbs 31 g

## 6.2 Greek-Style Salad

This classic Greek salad is easy to transport in a jar or closed container. It can also be made in a bowl at home.

Preparation time: 10 minutes

Cooking time: 0 minutes

Serving: 2

**Ingredients**

- ½ cucumber around 200 grams, halved lengthways and sliced

- 2 ripe tomatoes, each cut into eight pieces

- 100 grams feta, cut into small cubes

- ½ medium red onion, peeled and thinly sliced

- 50 grams pitted black olives (preferably Kalamata), drained

- 50 grams mixed salad leaves

**For the simple lemon dressing**

- 1 tablespoon fresh lemon juice

- 2 tablespoon extra-virgin olive oil

**Instructions**

Take a small bowl, combine together the lemon juice, olive oil, a pinch of sea salt, and enough crushed black pepper to make the dressing. Separate the dressing into two containers.

Top with the leaves and divide the cucumber, tomatoes, feta, onion, and olives between the containers. Until ready to toss, keep the leaves separated from the dressing at the bottom of the container. Refrigerate the container with the lid through until ready to eat. Start by giving the jar a good thrashing and eat the salad straight from it, or spoon it out onto a serving plate.

**Nutritional facts**

322 cals, Protein 10 g, Fats 27.5 g, Fiber 3.5 g, Carbs 6.5 g

# 6.3 Gut-friendly Chicory with Blue Cheese and Walnuts

The chicory and walnuts in this salad are high in soluble fiber, good for your gut. Soluble fiber, also known as a prebiotic, aids the production of important nutrients by gut bacteria in the colon and preserves the gut lining. This salad is a great appetizer that will assist in boosting digestion before the main course.

Preparation time: 10 minutes

Cooking time: 3 minutes

Serving: 2

## Ingredients

- 20g walnuts, roughly chopped

- 2 heads chicory, red or white

- Handful rocket, watercress and young spinach leaves

- 1 ripe pear around 125grams, quartered, cored and sliced

- 65g soft blue cheese, such as Roquefort

## For the cider vinegar dressing

- 1 teaspoon live cider vinegar

- 2 tablespoon extra-virgin olive oil

## Instructions

Toast the walnuts in a moderate non - stick frying pan for 2–3 minutes, until either golden brown in places, stirring the pan periodically. Allow drying on a board. Cut 6 thinly sliced from the chicory's root end, then split the leaves lengthwise, cutting those that are especially big in half. The leaves should be thoroughly cleaned and strained.

Arrange the chicory in a serving dish, and then top with the rocket and pear. Dot the cheese on top after cutting it into little pieces. Chop the walnuts coarsely and scatter them over the salad. Mix the vinegar and olive oil in a small mixing bowl, seasoning with sea salt and powdered black pepper to prepare the dressing. Toss the salad with the dressing before serving.

**Nutritional facts**

335 cals, Protein 9 g, Fats 29 g, Fiber 3 g, Carbs 8 g

---

# 6.4 Chicken, Bacon and Avocado Salad

The dressing's tiny bit of honey wonderfully balances the saltiness of the bacon.

Preparation time: 10 minutes

Cooking time: 4 minutes

Serving: 2

**Ingredients**

- 4 rashers streaky bacon
- 100g mixed salad leaves

- 10 cherry tomatoes cut in pieces

- 100g cooked chicken breast, sliced

- 1 medium avocado (stoned, peeled and sliced)

**For the mustard dressing**

- 2 tablespoon extra-virgin olive oil

- 1 teaspoon red or white wine vinegar

- 1 teaspoon Dijon mustard

- 1 teaspoon runny honey

**Instructions**

Take a small bowl, mix the oil, vinegar, mustard, and honey until slightly thickened to create the dressing. Season with a generous amount of ground black pepper and a pinch of sea salt.

Cook the bacon for about 2 minutes on each side in a small nonstick frying pan over medium heat or until crisp. Place to a cutting board and chop. Using two plates, divide the mixed leaves. Add the tomatoes, cut chicken, avocado, and bacon on the top. Just before serving, drizzle the mustard dressing over the salad and mix lightly.

**Nutritional facts**

495 cals, Protein 26 g, Fats 40 g, Fiber 5 g, Carbs 7 g

## 6.5 Chicken Tikka Salad

A delicious chicken salad that is perfect for a light meal.

Preparation time: 10 minutes

Cooking time: 8 minutes

Serving: 2

**Ingredients**

- 2 boneless, skinless chicken breasts (each around 175g), cut into roughly 3cm chunks

- 2 tablespoon full-fat live Greek yogurt

- 1 tablespoon tikka curry paste

- 1 tablespoon coconut or rapeseed oil

- 2 Little Gem lettuces, trimmed and leaves separated

- 2 medium tomatoes, roughly chopped

- ½ small red onion, peeled and finely chopped

- 2 tablespoon finely chopped fresh coriander leaves

- Fresh mint leaves (optional), to serve

- Lemon or lime wedges, to serve

**Instructions**

Combine the chicken, yogurt, and tikka paste in a mixing bowl. Mix everything thoroughly, then cover and chill for at least 1 hour, but preferably many hours or overnight.

Take a medium nonstick frying pan, heat the oil over medium-high heat. Season the chicken with a good teaspoon of salt and a generous amount of ground black pepper, then sauté for 6–8 minutes, frequently flipping until lightly browned and cooked through. If packing a lunch, set it aside to cool.

Divide the lettuce across two large basins or containers with lids.

Combine the tomatoes, onion, and coriander in a small bowl and season with salt and pepper. Toss the lettuce with spices.

Serve with lemon for squeezing over the chicken tikka pieces and mint leaves if using. If you're not going to consume it right away, keep it refrigerated.

**Nutritional facts**

315 cals, Protein 45 g, Fats 11 g, Fiber 3.5 g, Carbs 7.5 g

## 6.6 Chicken Caesar-Ish Salad

The mixed seeds here provide the crunch of croutons while being significantly more healthful.

Preparation time: 10 minutes

Cooking time: 3 minutes

Serving: 2

**Ingredients**

- 2 Little Gem lettuces, trimmed and leaves separated

- 12 cherry tomatoes, halved

- 200 grams cooked chicken breast, cut or shredded into small pieces

- 10 grams mixed seeds

- 20 grams Parmesan, finely grated

**For the yogurt dressing**

- 75g Greek yogurt

- ½ small garlic clove, peeled and crushed

- Pinch dried mixed herbs

- 1 tbsp. extra-virgin olive oil

**Instructions**

In a mixing dish, combine the yogurt, garlic, herbs, oil, and 2 tablespoons cold water to make the dressing. Toss with a pinch of salt and a generous amount of freshly ground black pepper.

Drain the lettuce thoroughly after washing it. Distribute the leaves among two shallow dishes or closed containers, then top with the tomatoes. Put the chicken on top, then drizzle with the dressing and sprinkle with the mixed seeds and Parmesan. Serve with freshly ground black pepper.

**Nutritional facts**

300 cals, Protein 32 g, Fats 16 g, Fiber 2 g, Carbs 5.5 g

# 6.7 Salmon Salad Bowl

Serve the salad warm as a substantial lunch or supper, or store it in a covered container for a nutritious packed meal.

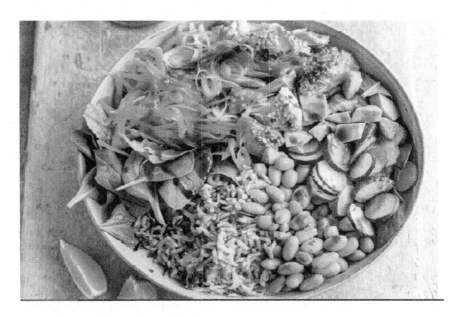

Preparation time: 10 minutes

Cooking time: 32 minutes

Serving: 2

**Ingredients**

- 25 grams whole grain brown rice, or brown and wild rice mix

- 75 grams freeze edamame beans or peas

- 120 grams salmon fillets

- 1 teaspoon sesame seeds

- Pinch crushed dried chili

- 2 large handfuls of spinach leaves or baby salad leaves

- ½ medium avocado, stoned, peeled and chopped

- 1 medium carrot coarsely grated

- 2 spring onions finely sliced

- 4 radishes sliced

- Lime wedges to serve

**For the soy and lime dressing**

- 2 tablespoon dark soy sauce

- 1 tablespoon sesame oil

- 1 teaspoon fresh lime juice

- 1 teaspoon runny honey

## Instructions

Preheated oven to 200 °C and line a small baking pan with foil. Bring a small pot half-filled with water to a boil a little bit. Cook till the rice is softened. Bring the edamame beans or peas back to a boil while stirring. As quickly as possible, drain.

Combine the soya sauce, sesame oil, lime juice, and honey in a separate bowl to create the dressing.

Drizzle 2 tablespoons of the filling over the salmon on the prepared tray, skin-side down. Top with sesame seeds and chili flakes, if preferred. Bake the chicken until it is just cooked through. (When a fork is inserted into the salmon, it should readily flake into big pieces.) Split the herbs, rice, and lentils or peas into two bowls. Alongside the greens, arrange the avocado, carrot, spring onions, and radishes. Serve with lime pieces to squeeze over, then flake the salmon into the bowl. Drizzle with the remaining dressing.

**Nutritional facts**

542 cals, Protein 33 g, Fats 35.5 g, Fiber 6 g, Carbs 20g

## 6.8 Edamame and Tuna Salad

Edamame beans have protein and fiber, are a terrific addition to any salad. The crisp, green snap of these flexible young beans is appealing.

Preparation time: 5 minutes

Cooking time: 1 minute

Serving: 2

**Ingredients**

- 200g frozen edamame beans
- 2 spring onions, trimmed and thinly sliced
- 110g can no-drain tuna steak in olive oil
- 15g fresh flat-leaf parsley or coriander, leaves roughly chopped
- 1½ tablespoon live cider vinegar
- 3 tablespoon extra-virgin olive oil
- 2 large handfuls rocket or mixed leaves

**Instructions**

Fill a heatproof bowl halfway with edamame beans and top with just-boiled water from a kettle. Stir and set aside for 1 minute to let the beans defrost (cooking isn't necessary). Drain and rinse well with cold water.

Combine the beans, spring onions, tuna, and herbs in a mixing dish, then break the tuna into flakes with a fork. Toss the salad with vinegar and olive oil, season with sea salt and plenty of ground black pepper, and toss thoroughly. Just before serving, fold in the leaves.

**Nutritional facts**

408 cals, Protein 26 g, Fats 27 g, Fiber 5 g, Carbs 12 g

# 6.9 Crab, Courgette and Avocado Salad

This fantastic summer salad is packed with nutrients, including selenium and iodine, which can be deficient in our diets.

Preparation time: 5 minutes

Cooking time: 2 minutes

Serving: 2

**Ingredients**

- 20g pine nuts

- 2 medium courgette (each around 250g), trimmed

- 1 small avocado, stoned, peeled and diced

- 2 large handfuls rocket

- 100g white crabmeat, tinned or fresh

- 1 red chili, thinly sliced or diced (optional)

**For the lime dressing**

- 3 tablespoon extra-virgin olive oil

- 1 tablespoon fresh lime juice

- ½ teaspoon wholegrain mustard

- 1 tablespoon finely chopped fresh mint

**Instructions**

Mix the olive oil, lime juice, mustard, and mint in a small bowl to create the dressing.

Scatter the pine nuts and toast for 1–2 minutes, tossing periodically until lightly toasted in a small frying pan. Place the mixture on a platter and put it aside.

Slice the courgette into long, wide strips and place them in a large mixing basin using a vegetable peeler. Tossed with salt and black pepper and tossed lightly with the avocado and rocket leaves. Scatter the crabmeat on top, followed by the pine nuts and, if desired, the chili. To serve, drizzle with the dressing.

**Nutritional facts**

421 cals, Protein 16.5 g, Fats 36.5 g, Fiber 5 g, Carbs 4 g

## 6.10 Tuna Salad

Cauliflower replaces the typical potatoes in this classic salad with a low-carb twist.

Preparation time: 5 minutes

Cooking time: 8 minute

Serving: 2

**Ingredients**

- 100g green beans, trimmed and halved

- 100g cauliflower, cut into small florets

- 2 medium eggs, fridge cold

- 50g mixed salad leaves

- 8 cherry tomatoes, halved

- 110g can no-drain tuna steak in olive oil

- 30g canned anchovies in oil, drained

- 40g pitted black or green olives

**For the creamy, garlicky yogurt dressing**

- 1 tablespoon extra-virgin olive oil

- 50g full-fat live Greek yogurt

- ½ small garlic clove, peeled and crushed

## Instructions

In a separate bowl, mix the oil, garlic, and 2 tablespoons cold water to make the dressing. Add a pinch of salt and black pepper to taste.

Fill a small saucepan halfway with water and bring to a boil. Return to fire and simmer for 3 minutes with the beans and cauliflower florets. With a slotted spoon, lift out the chicken and place it in a bowl of cool water. Bring the water back to a boil. Cook for 8 minutes after adding the eggs. With a slotted spoon, lift out the eggs and place them in a separate bowl of frigid water. Drain the green beans and cauliflower well, and then combine them with the mixed leaves and tomatoes on two plates.

Peel the eggs, quarter them, and toss them with tuna flakes, anchovies, and olives in a salad. Just before serving, drizzle with the dressing.

## Nutritional facts

362 cals, Protein 30 g, Fats 23 g, Fiber 4.5 g, Carbs 7 g

## 6.11 Homemade coleslaw

A crisp and colorful salad that is high in fiber and may be served with any meal.

Preparation time: 5 minutes

Cooking time: 0 minute

Serving: 4

## Ingredients

- 100g live, full-fat yoghurt, preferably Greek

- 100g mayonnaise of good quality

- 14 cup red cabbage (medium) (around 200g)

- 1 medium carrot, cut into long, thin shreds after trimming and coarsely grating

- 2 trimmed and thinly sliced spring onions

- 1 clipped and thinly cut celery stick (optional)

## Instructions

Take a large mixing bowl, combine the yogurt, mayonnaise, and 2 tablespoons cold water, along with a pinch of black pepper. Remove any damaged outer leaves and the rigid center core from the cabbage. Add the cabbage to the yogurt dressing after shredding it as finely as possible. If used, toss together the carrots, spring onions, and celery in a large mixing basin.

## Nutritional facts

251 cals, Protein 2.5 g, Fats 24 g, Fiber 2.5 g, Carbs 5 g

# Chapter 7 Occasional Treats

## 7.1 Apple Crisp with Cinnamon

These tasty treats are high in soluble fiber, which is good for you. Best served as a bit of dessert after a meal.

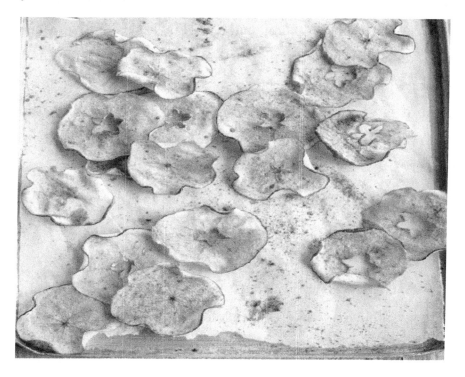

Preparation time: 35 minutes

Cooking time: 5 hours

Serving: 2

### Ingredients

- 2 tablespoons coconut oil

- 12 tsp cinnamon powder

- 1 red-skinned apple, big (around 200g)

## Instructions

Oven preheated to 130°C. The nonstick baking paper should be used to line a big baking pan. Melt the coconut oil with the cinnamon over low heat and put it aside in a small saucepan. Remove the apple's top, tail, and core. Finely slice into 3–4mm thick discs. Spritz the apple slices with the cinnamon oil and arrange them in a single layer on the baking pan. Bake for a total of 112 hours or until extremely dry and crisp. Turn the oven off and let the apples dehydrate for another 2–3 hours. To serve, divide the mixture between two individuals.

## Nutritional Facts

81 cals, Protein 0.6 g, Fats 3.5 g, Fiber 1 g, Carbs 11 g

## 7.2 Almond and Orange Loaf

A zesty, delicious cake. It's incredible since it's made using whole oranges that don't need to be peeled. Serve in thin slices while still heated

Preparation time: 30 minutes

Cook time: 1 hour

Servings: 10

## Ingredients

- 2 medium oranges (about 150g each), cleaned

- 8 dates with soft pits

- 4 tbsp extra virgin olive oil

- 4 eggs (medium)

- 300 g almonds, ground

- 12 tablespoons baking powder

- 15 g almond flake

## Instructions

Prick each orange with the point of a knife 20 times and put it in a microwave-safe bowl. Microwave on high for 10 minutes, until either very soft, covered with a plate. Set the oven to 190 degrees Celsius. The non-stick baking paper should line the bottom and sides of a 900g loaf pan. Allow the oranges to cool completely before cutting in half and removing any seeds. In a food processor, whizz the oranges and dates with olive oil and eggs until well combined. Blend in the powdered almonds, baking powder, and 4 tablespoons water until a thick batter forms. Pour the batter into the greased tin, distributing it out to the edges. Bake for 40–45 minutes, until either nicely browned or stiff to the touch or until risen golden brown and firm to the touch. Chill for 30 minutes in the pan before turning out and cutting into thin strips to serve.

## Nutritional Facts

326 cals, Protein 12 g, Fats 24 g, Fiber 1.5 g, Carbs 14.5 g

# 7.3 Parsnip and Ginger Tray bake

This tray bake is buttery and flavorful, with sweet ginger bursts.

Preparation time: 45 minutes

Cook time: 2 hours

Servings: 16

## Ingredients

- 150 g coconut oil + a little more for frying

- 3 eggs (big)

- 50 grams pitted soft dates, halved

- 4 teaspoons ginger powder

- 1 teaspoon cinnamon or cardamom powder

- 1 teaspoon nutmeg powder

- 1 teaspoon extract de Vanilla

- 250 grams peeled and finely shredded parsnips (probably 2 medium)

- 100g plain whole meal flour

- 2 teaspoons of baking powder

- 2 stem ginger balls (about 30 grams), soaked and roughly cut into 1cm pieces

## Instructions

Oven preheated to 190 degrees Celsius. The non-stick baking paper should be used to line the base and sides of a 20cm flat square cake pan. In a food processor, blend the eggs, coconut oil or butter, dates, fresh ginger, cardamom or cinnamon, nutmeg, and vanilla until thoroughly incorporated. Blitz again on the pulse setting with the parsnips, flour, and baking powder till the dough comes together again and forms a soft crumb. Pour into the greased tin and distribute to the edges. Dot the stem ginger pieces into the batter and softly push them in. Baked for 40–45 minutes, until either golden brown or slightly risen. Allow 10 minutes for the cake to settle in the pan before transferring to a cooling rack ultimately. Serve warm or cold, cut into 16 squares.

## Nutritional Facts

151 cals, Protein 3 g, Fats 11 g, Fiber 2 g, CARBS 9 g

## 7.4 Mango Fruit Pots

A delectable delicacy with a tropical flavor.

Preparation time: 15 minutes

Cook time: 20 minutes

Serving: 4

## Ingredients

- 10 grams desiccated coconut, unsweetened

- 2 halved passion fruits

- 1 peeled, stoned, and chopped small ripe mango (about 300 grams).

- 1/2 tiny limes, coarsely grated (optional).

- Yogurt made with coconut milk, 300 grams, thoroughly chilled

## Instructions

Toast the coconut for 2–3 minutes over medium heat in a small saucepan, stirring often. Allow cooling. Push the desired fruit out of the hulls using a teaspoon and arrange in a dish. Stir in the mango and, if using, the lime zest. Start dividing the mango and passion fruit among four porcelain cups or dessert plates, reserving a little amount for garnish. Finish with the roasted coconut and saved mango combination, followed by the yogurt.

## Nutritional Facts

207cals, Protein 3 g, Fats 16 g, Fiber 3.5 g, Carbs 11 g

# 7.5 Chocolate Mug Cake

For immediate gooey chocolate delight, try this.

Preparation time: 25 minutes

Cook time: 40inutes

Servings: 2

## Ingredients

- 1 tablespoon of coconut oil

- 4 coarsely chopped soft pitted dates about 30 grams

- 1 medium egg, properly beaten

- Ground almonds, 25 grams

- Cocoa powder 7 grams (around 1 tbsp).

- 1/4 teaspoon baking powder

- 1 plain dark chocolate square about 5 grams around 85 percent cocoa solids

- Serve with a handful of fresh raspberries.

- A microwave-safe cup is required to hold around 300ml.

## Instructions

Stir the coconut oil in the cup for a few seconds on high in the microwave. Allowing it to overheat is not a good idea. In a cup, incorporate the dates, egg, almonds, cocoa powder, baking powder, and a tiny amount of flaked sea salt with a fork until thoroughly blended. If necessary, add an additional 1–2 tablespoons of water to lighten the mixture. Microwave on high for approximately 1 minute, just until the cake has risen, solid, and just starting to retract from the edges of the mug, pressing the square of chocolate straight into the surface of the cake batter until immersed. Turn the cake out onto a platter, carefully hold the hot cup, and cut it half to expose the melted chocolate. Divide into two dishes and top with a couple of fresh raspberries on each half.

**Nutritional Facts**

216 cals, Protein 8 g, Fats 17 g, Fiber 1 g, Carbs 7.5 g

## 7.6 Raisin and Almond Chocolate Pennies

These little chocolate treats are packed with healthy polyphenols that your gut bacteria will enjoy, so go for dark chocolate with 85 percent cocoa contents. The almonds provide protein and crunch, while the raisins give flavor and additional fiber.

Preparation time: 30 minutes

Cook time: 45 minutes

Servings: 20

**Ingredients**

- 100 grams dark chocolate (plain) (around 85 percent cocoa solids)

- 25 g flaked almonds, roasted

- 25 grams of raisins

## Instructions

The non-stick baking paper should be used to line a baking pan. Split the chocolate into blocks and put in a heatproof bowl set over a pan of gently boiling salted water, ensuring that the bowl's base does not contact the water's surface. Allow for a 5-minute gradual melting period, stirring periodically. Microwave for 1–2 minutes at high temperature, or until nearly completely melted, then whisk. Allowing the chocolate to overheat will cause it to harden or burn. Remove the heated bowl from the pan with care and, to use a teaspoon, spoon 20 spoonfuls of melted chocolate onto the tray to space them evenly. On the topping of the melted chocolate, distribute the almonds and raisins. Allow for a couple of hours of setting time. Gently pry the pennies off the baking paper with a knife. Area in a closed jar and keep in a cool place for close to a week.

## Nutritional Facts

38 cals, Protein 0.5 g, Fats 2 g, Fiber 0 g, Carbs 4 g

## 7.7 Bay Byron Bars

A delicious, crispy snack that will offer you a jolt of energy and lots of fiber. These bars aren't as sweet as store-bought versions.

Preparation time: 30 minutes

Cooking time: 1 hour 35 minutes

Servings: 16

## Ingredients

- coconut oil 125 grams

- 150 grams of giant oats

- 100 grams flaked almonds, roasted

- Flax seeds 25 grams (linseeds)

- 2 medium egg whites

- 75 grams dried cranberries, coarsely chopped

- 2 tablespoons extract de Vanilla

## Instructions

Oven preheated to 200 degrees. The non-stick baking paper should be used to line the foundation of a 20cm loose-based square cake pan. Take a saucepan over low heat, melt the coconut oil. Remove from the heat and whisk in the oats, almonds, flax seeds, cranberries, and a sprinkle of sea salt until well combined. Scramble together the egg whites until they are somewhat foamy. Combine with the oat mixture and stir thoroughly. Fill the prepared pan halfway with the mixture and smooth the top with the slotted spoon, pushing down firmly to compact all ingredients. 15–18 minutes in the oven, or until gently browned. Give for at least 1 hour of cooling time in the tin before cutting into slender bars.

**Nutritional Facts**

170 cals, Protein 3 g, Fats 12.5 g, Fiber 1.9 g, Carbs 10 g

# 7.8 Fudgy Chocolate Bars

No-bake bars that are extremely rich and include a lot of fiber, making them a fantastic alternative to sweet confectionary. It's a once-in-a-while treat that's best enjoyed after a meal.

Preparation time: 1 hour

Cooking time: 0 minutes

Serving: 20

## Ingredients

- 150 grams mixed nuts (roughly chopped)
- 150 grams soft pitted prunes (quartered)
- 150 grams ready-to-eat dried apricots (quartered)
- 50 grams coconut oil (not melted)
- 25 grams cocoa powder

## Instructions

Cover the sides of a 900g loaf tin with cling film, leaving plenty of overhang. In a food processor, blitz the nuts until finely chopped but not crushed. Pour into a mixing basin. Blend the prunes and apricots together in a food processor until a thick mixture forms.

Add the cocoa powder and coconut oil to the nuts in the food processor. Blend until the mixture comes together to form a rough ball. Pour into the prepared tin and distribute to the edges. Cover the chocolate mixture with the cling film that hangs over the edge. Freeze it for 1 hour, or till it completely solid.

Remove the frozen item from the freezer, unwrap it, and place it on a cutting board. Cut the dough into 20 1cm bars. To keep the bars from sticking together, layer them in a covered container with baking paper sheets. Refrigerate for up to 2 weeks.

**Nutritional facts**

101cals, Protein 3 g, Fats 6.5 g, Fiber 1.5 g, Carbs 7 g

## 7.9 Strawberry and Vanilla Yoghurt

A quick and easy yoghurt that can be served as a treat or brunch. Strawberries are naturally delicious, yet they have a modest sugar content.

Preparation time: 10 minutes

Cooking time: 0 minutes

Serving: 4

**Ingredients**

250g fresh strawberries (hulled and halved)

½ teaspoon vanilla extract

300g full-fat live Greek yoghurt

## Instructions

Mash the strawberries in a mixing dish to release their juices and crush the berries. In a second bowl, combine the yoghurt and vanilla extract, then gently mix in the strawberries. Keep cold by dividing across small dishes or glasses.

## Nutritional facts

123 cals, Protein 4.5 g, Fats 8 g, Fiber 2.5 g, Carbs 7 g

## 7.10 Chocolate Beetroot Brownies

Anyone can guess what the primary ingredient is!

Preparation time: 20 minutes

Cooking time: 20 minutes

Serving: 20

## Ingredients

- 3 large eggs
- 60g Choco powder
- 100 grams coconut oil plus extra for greasing
- 275 grams cooked beetroot washed and cut into small portions
- 100 grams soft dates
- 100 grams whole meal self-rising flour

- 1 teaspoon cinnamon

- 1 teaspoon bicarbonate of soda

- 75 grams plain dark chocolate (around 85% cocoa solids), roughly chopped

**Instructions**

Preheat the oven to 200°C. Non-stick baking paper should be used to line the base and sides of a 20cm loose-based square cake tin. In a food processor, add the beets, eggs, chocolate powder, dates, and coconut oil and pulse until smooth. You can also use a hand mixer to blend the ingredients in a bowl.

Blend in the flour, cinnamon, a pinch of sea salt, and bicarbonate of soda until smooth. If necessary, add an extra tablespoon of water to loosen the mixture. Stir in the chocolate, then spoon into the prepared tin, spreading evenly. Bake for 20 minutes, or till the dough has risen and is firm to the touch. Wait for 10 minutes to cool in the tin before turning out and cutting into squares to serve.

**Nutritional facts**

128cals, Protein 3 g, Fats 8 g, Fiber 1.5 g, Carbs 10.5 g

## 7.10 Seeded Whole meal Bread

This is a wonderful loaf that is somewhat chewy. Slices can be frozen if they aren't used right away. It's perfect for a bread maker.

Preparation time: 20 minutes

Cooking time: 20 minutes

Serving: 20

## Ingredients

- 7g sachet dried fast-action yeast

- 425 grams strong whole meal bread flour + 1 tablespoon extra for kneading

- 100g mixed seeds

- 2 tablespoon skimmed milk powder

- 1 tablespoon soft light brown sugar

- 1½ teaspoon fine sea salt

- 1 tablespoon olive oil and some more for extra greasing

## Instructions

Take a large mixing bowl, combine the yeast, flour, seeds, milk powder, sugar, and salt, and create a well in the center. To make 350ml lukewarm water, fill a jug halfway with 150ml just-boiled water from a kettle and the other half with 200ml cold water.

Pour in the oil into the flour mixture. Mix every ingredients together with a large spoon until it forms a rough ball.

Knead the dough for 5 minutes on a lightly floured surface. The dough will be gooey, so sprinkle the surface with flour if required. Seal with cling wrap and place in a lightly greased basin, and set aside for 112–2 hours, or until about doubled in size. Gather the dough and roll it into a ball with your hands. Place the dough on top of a baking tray lined with baking paper. Make an 18cm round out of the dough. Leave to prove for 1–112 hours, or until well risen, after scoring three times with a sharp knife.

Preheated the oven to 220. Bake for 25 minutes, or till it gets golden brown, after removing the cling wrap. When you touch the base, it should sound hollow. Allow to cool on a wire rack. Serve thinly sliced (about 65g per serving).

## Nutritional facts

178 cals, Protein 6.5 g, Fats 4 g, Fiber 4 g, Carbs 27.5 g

# Conclusion

Intermittent fasting entails going without food either completely or partially before eating normally again.

You won't have to starve yourself if you practice intermittent fasting, sometimes known as Intermittent Fasting. It also doesn't permit you to eat a lot of unhealthy food while you aren't fasting. Instead of eating meals and snacks throughout the day, you eat within a set period.

Intermittent fasting has survived the test of time and, in addition to weight loss, has been demonstrated to have a variety of health benefits. Women over 50 may benefit from intermittent fasting to lose weight and reduce their risk of acquiring age-related disorders. According to a new study by Baylor College of Medicine, intermittent fasting can lower blood pressure. Fasting decreases blood pressure via altering the gut microbiota, according to the study.

Intermittent fasting advocates believe that it is simpler to stick to than typical calorie-controlled diets. Intermittent fasting is a personal experience for each person, and different approaches will suit different people.

Of course, many women over 50 are concerned about losing weight and trying to improve their health. Lower metabolism, achy joints, diminished muscle mass, and even sleep troubles make it more difficult to lose weight beyond 50. Simultaneously, decreasing fat, particularly harmful belly fat, can significantly lower your chance of serious health problems, including diabetes, heart attacks, and cancer.

As you become older, your chances of contracting a variety of ailments rise. When it comes to weight loss and reducing the risk of acquiring age-related disorders, intermittent fasting for women over 50 may be a virtual fountain of youth in some circumstances.

Some people claim that IF has helped them lose weight simply because the limited eating window forces them to eat fewer calories. For example, instead of three meals and two snacks, they may only have time for two meals and one snack. They become more conscious of their foods and avoid processed carbohydrates, bad fats, and empty calories.

Intermittent fasting does more than burn fat, according to research. Changes in this metabolic switch affect the body and the brain, Mattson explains. Mattson's study appeared in the New England Journal of Medicine, and it detailed several health benefits associated with the practice. Among them include longer life, a thinner body, and a sharper mind. "During intermittent fasting, various things happen that protect organs from any severe diseases including age-related neurological disorders, type 2 diabetes, heart disease, even inflammatory bowel disease and many malignancies," he explains.

Intermittent fasting improves working memory in animals and verbal memory in adults, according to research. Fasting for a short period improved blood pressure, resting heart rates, and other heart-related parameters. This book has all the recipes you will need and will help you in achieving your goal. The recipes are provided easily and also for beginners. Women over 50 can use these recipes easily, and this book is all they need. There is no such thing as a one-size-fits-all method to dieting. That holds for intermittent fasting as well. Women should, on average, adopt a more relaxed attitude to fasting than males. Shorter fasting times, fewer fasting days, and taking a lower number of calories on fasting days are all possible options.

# 28 DAYS MEAL PLAN

| | 1st Day Plan |
|---|---|
| Breakfast | Chocolate Granola |
| Lunch | Creamy Mushroom Soup |
| Snack | Ice Berry Shake |
| Dinner | Lamb Saag |
| Dessert | Strawberry and Vanilla Yoghurt |
| | 2nd Day Plan |
| Breakfast | Instant Porridge Cup |
| Lunch | Instant Noodle Soup |
| Snack | Ginger Shake |
| Dinner | Smocked Haddock with Lentils |
| Dessert | Fudgy Chocolate Bars |
| | 3rd Day Plan |
| Breakfast | Banana and Pecan Muffin |
| Lunch | Easy Chicken Tagine |
| Snack | Apple Crisp with Cinnamon |
| Dinner | Beef Rending |
| Dessert | Ice Berry Shake |
| | 4th Day Plan |
| Breakfast | Blueberry Pancakes |
| Lunch | Sausages with Onion Gravy and Cauliflower Mash |
| Snack | Mango Fruit Pots |
| Dinner | Mediterranean Fish Bake |
| Dessert | Chai Smoothie |
| | 5th Day Plan |
| Breakfast | Citrus Salad |
| Lunch | Cheat's One-Pot Cassoulet |
| Snack | Chocolate Mug Cake |
| Dinner | Pie with Swede Mash |
| Dessert | Mango Fruit Pots |

| | 6<sup>th</sup> Day Plan |
|---|---|

| | **6<sup>th</sup> Day Plan** |
|---|---|
| Breakfast | Warm Berry with Yoghurt |
| Lunch | Chicken and Pea Soup |
| Snack | Gazpacho Shake |
| Dinner | Salmon Salad Bowl |
| Dessert | Almond and Orange Loaf |
| | **7<sup>th</sup> Day Plan** |
| Breakfast | Smoked Salmon Omelet |
| Lunch | Pan-Fried Pork with Apple and Leak |
| Snack | Almond and Orange Loaf |
| Dinner | Chicken Caesar-Ish Salad |
| Dessert | Strawberry and Vanilla Yoghurt |
| | **8<sup>th</sup> Day Plan** |
| Breakfast | Turmeric Boost Breakfast |
| Lunch | Satay Chicken |
| Snack | Parsnip and Ginger Tray Bake |
| Dinner | Mussels with Creamy Tarragon Sauce |
| Dessert | Fudgy Chocolate Bars |
| | **9<sup>th</sup> Day Plan** |
| Breakfast | Pear and Cinnamon Porridge |
| Lunch | Tomato Soup |
| Snack | Banana Nutty Shake |
| Dinner | Greek-Style Salad |
| Dessert | Ice Berry Shake |
| | **10<sup>th</sup> Day Plan** |
| Breakfast | Overnight Oats |
| Lunch | Broccoli Cheese Soup |
| Snack | Cashew, Carrot, and Orange Shake |
| Dinner | Baked Salmon with Pea and Broccoli Mash |
| Dessert | Strawberry and Chocolate Shake |
| | **11<sup>th</sup> Day Plan** |
| Breakfast | Sliced Avocado on Toast |
| Lunch | Lamb Chops with Minted Peas and Feta |
| Snack | Apple Crisp with Cinnamon |

| Dinner | Lamb Saag |
| --- | --- |
| Dessert | Banana Nutty Shake |
| **12th Day Plan** | |
| Breakfast | Citrus Yogurt Parfait |
| Lunch | Parma Pork |
| Snack | Fudgy Chocolate Bars |
| Dinner | Smocked Haddock with Lentils |
| Dessert | Strawberry and Chocolate Shake |
| **13th Day Plan** | |
| Breakfast | Peanut Butter Oatmeal balls |
| Lunch | Easy Jerk Chicken |
| Snack | Raisin and Almond Chocolate Pennies |
| Dinner | Speedy Pizza |
| Dessert | Mango Fruit Pots |
| **14th Day Plan** | |
| Breakfast | Blueberry Pancakes |
| Lunch | Peppered Pork Stir-Fry |
| Snack | Bay Byron Bars |
| Dinner | Thai Curry with Prawns |
| Dessert | Almond and Orange Loaf |
| **15th Day Plan** | |
| Breakfast | Chocolate Granola |
| Lunch | Courgetti Spaghetti with Nuts, Spinach and Pancetta |
| Snack | Chocolate Mug Cake |
| Dinner | Pie with Swede Mash |
| Dessert | Parsnip and Ginger Tray Bake |
| **16th Day Plan** | |
| Breakfast | Scrambled Eggs with Mushrooms and Spinach |
| Lunch | Satay Chicken |
| Snack | Seeded Whole meal Bread |
| Dinner | Chicken Caesar-Ish Salad |
| Dessert | Apple Crisp with Cinnamon |
| **17th Day Plan** | |
| Breakfast | Banana and Pecan Muffin |

| Lunch | Roast Chicken Thighs with Lemon |
|---|---|
| Snack | Minted Cucumber and Avocado Shake |
| Dinner | Tuna Salad |
| Dessert | Strawberry and Vanilla Yoghurt |
| | 18th Day Plan |
| Breakfast | Baked Beans |
| Lunch | Chicken, Pepper and Chorizo Bake |
| Snack | Raisin and Almond Chocolate Pennies |
| Dinner | Greek-Style Salad |
| Dessert | Bay Byron Bars |
| | 19th Day Plan |
| Breakfast | Breakfast Plums |
| Lunch | Chicken Tikka Masala |
| Snack | Parsnip and Ginger Tray Bake |
| Dinner | Lamb Saag |
| Dessert | Fudgy Chocolate Bars |
| | 20th Day Plan |
| Breakfast | Mushrooms on Toasted Sourdough |
| Lunch | One-pot Roast Chicken |
| Snack | Chai Smoothie |
| Dinner | Beef Rending |
| Dessert | Seeded Whole meal Bread |
| | 21st Day Plan |
| Breakfast | Warm Berry with Yoghurt |
| Lunch | Turkey Fajitas |
| Snack | Strawberry and Chocolate Shake |
| Dinner | Salmon Salad Bowl |
| Dessert | Strawberry and Vanilla Yoghurt |
| | 22nd Day Plan |
| Breakfast | Plantain Chips |
| Lunch | Simple Chicken Casserole |
| Snack | Mango Fruit Pots |
| Dinner | Quinoa, Broccoli and Asparagus Salad |
| Dessert | Bay Byron Bars |

| | 23rd Day Plan |
|---|---|
| Breakfast | Glazed Dried Fruit and Nuts |
| Lunch | Chinese-Style Drumsticks |
| Snack | Apple Crisp with Cinnamon |
| Dinner | Sesame Salmon with Broccoli and Tomatoes |
| Dessert | Raisin and Almond Chocolate Pennies |
| | 24th Day Plan |
| Breakfast | Sweet and Spicy Roasted Nuts |
| Lunch | Chicken Goujons with Parmesan Crumb |
| Snack | Ice Berry Shake |
| Dinner | Chicken Tikka Salad |
| Dessert | Banana Nutty Shake |
| | 25th Day Plan |
| Breakfast | Smoked Salmon Omelet |
| Lunch | Chicken Wrapped in Parma Ham |
| Snack | Almond and Orange Loaf |
| Dinner | Baked Salmon with Pea and Broccoli Mash |
| Dessert | Chocolate Mug Cake |
| | 26th Day Plan |
| Breakfast | Citrus Yogurt Parfait |
| Lunch | Easy Chicken Tagine |
| Snack | Secded Whole meal Bread |
| Dinner | Tuna Salad |
| Dessert | Bay Byron Bars |
| | 27th Day Plan |
| Breakfast | Instant Porridge Cup |
| Lunch | Chicken Tikka Masala |
| Snack | Parsnip and Ginger Tray Bake |
| Dinner | Speedy Pizza |
| Dessert | Raisin and Almond Chocolate Pennies |
| | 28th Day Plan |
| Breakfast | Sliced Avocado on Toast |

| Lunch | Perfect Pulled Pork |
| --- | --- |
| Snack | Bay Byron Bars |
| Dinner | Mediterranean Fish Bake |
| Dessert | Apple Crisp with Cinnamon |

Made in the USA
Monee, IL
27 April 2022